THE AMERICAN HEART ASSOCIATION BLOOD PRESSURE LOWERING DIET COOKBOOK

Reducing Hypertension And Excess Weight Through Eating A Simple, Easy And Delicious Low Salt Meals

BY
WILFORD J. WARNER

COPYRIGHT

TABLE OF CONTENTS

INTRODUCTION I

WHAT IS BLOOD PRESSURE?

Blood pressure is the force exerted by the blood on the walls of the arteries as it flows through them. This force is generated by the pumping action of the heart, which creates a pressure gradient that drives the blood flow.

The two numbers that represent blood pressure, systolic and diastolic, correspond to different phases of the heart's pumping cycle. During systole, the heart contracts to push blood out into the arteries, which causes an increase in blood pressure. The maximum pressure exerted by the blood during this phase is the systolic pressure.

During diastole, the heart relaxes and refills with blood, which causes a decrease in blood pressure. The minimum pressure exerted by the blood during this phase is diastolic.

The measurement of blood pressure is influenced by several factors, including the amount of blood pumped by the heart, the resistance of the arteries, and the elasticity of the arterial walls. These factors can be affected by various physiological processes, such as the release of hormones, the activity of the nervous system, and the contraction of smooth muscle in the arterial walls.

High blood pressure (hypertension) occurs when the force of the blood against the arterial walls is consistently too high. This can cause damage to the arteries and increase the risk of cardiovascular disease. Low blood pressure (hypotension) occurs when the force of the blood against the arterial walls is consistently too low, which can lead to symptoms such as dizziness and fainting.

UNDERSTANDING HYPERTENSION

Hypertension, commonly referred to as high blood pressure, is a condition in which the force of blood against the walls of the arteries is consistently too high. Blood pressure is measured using two numbers, systolic (the pressure when the heart beats) and diastolic (the pressure when the heart is at rest between beats), expressed in millimeters of mercury (mmHg). A normal blood pressure reading is around 120/80 mmHg.

TYPES OF HYPERTENSION:

Primary Hypertension: This is the most common type of hypertension, and it has no known cause. Primary hypertension is often related to lifestyle factors such as a diet high in salt, alcohol consumption, smoking, physical inactivity, and obesity.

Secondary hypertension: This type of hypertension is caused by an underlying medical condition, such as kidney disease, sleep apnea, thyroid problems, or certain medications.

Hypertension is a major risk factor for cardiovascular disease, including heart attack, stroke, and heart failure. It can also damage the blood vessels in the kidneys, eyes, and brain, leading to kidney disease, vision problems, and cognitive decline.

Symptoms of hypertension are usually not present until the condition has progressed to a severe stage. Therefore, hypertension is often referred to as a "silent killer" and it is important to regularly monitor blood pressure.

Treatment for hypertension typically involves lifestyle changes such as exercise, weight loss, a healthy diet (e.g. low in sodium), and limiting alcohol and tobacco use. Medications, such as diuretics, ACE inhibitors, angiotensin receptor blockers (ARBs), calcium channel blockers, and beta-blockers, may also be prescribed to manage hypertension.

KEY COMPONENTS OF A BLOOD PRESSURE DIET

There are certain foods to Avoid when trying to Lower Blood Pressure

Avoiding over-processed foods, such as deli meat and canned soups, in favor of nutrient-rich whole foods, may help you manage your blood pressure.

Diet can have a big impact on your blood pressure, which is the force of your blood against the walls of your blood vessels.

Salty foods in particular can cause high blood pressure. When you eat salt, your body retains more fluids, raising your blood volume and pressure. Sugary foods and foods that are high in saturated fats can also increase blood pressure.

Whether or not you follow a particular diet, certain foods and ingredients may raise your blood pressure or help keep it high. Limiting these foods may help manage your blood pressure.

SALT, OR SPECIFICALLY THE SODIUM IN SALT, is a major contributor to high blood pressure and heart disease. This is because of how it affects fluid balance in the blood.

Table salt is around 40 percent sodium. Some amount of salt is important for health, but it's easy to eat too much. The AHA recommends getting no more than 2,300 mg of sodium — the equivalent of 1 teaspoon of salt — each day.

Most of the sodium in the American diet comes from packaged, processed food rather than what you add to the table.

Sodium may be hidden in unexpected places.

The following foods, known as the "salty six," are major contributors to people's daily salt intake:

- **BREAD AND ROLLS**
- **PIZZA**
- **SANDWICHES**
- **COLD CUTS AND CURED MEATS**
- **CANNED SOUP**
- **BURRITOS AND TACOS**
- **DELI MEAT**

PROCESSED DELI AND LUNCH MEATS are often packed with sodium. That's because manufacturers cure, season, and preserve these meats with salt.

According to our research database, just two slices of bologna contain 910 mg of sodium. One frankfurter, or hot dog, contains 567 mg.

Adding other high-salt foods, such as bread, cheese, various condiments, and pickles, means that a sandwich can easily become very high in sodium.

FROZEN PIZZA
The combination of INGREDIENTS in frozen pizzas means they're high in sugar, saturated fat, and sodium. Frozen pizza can have especially high levels of sodium.

CHEESE is often high in sodium. Just two slices of American cheese contain 512 mg of sodium. This is generally in combination with salty or sugary pizza dough and crust, cured meats, and tomato sauce.

To maintain flavor in the pizza once it's been cooked, manufacturers often add a lot of salt.

One 12-inch pepperoni pizza, cooked from frozen, contains 3,140 sodium, which is well above the daily limit of 2,300 mg.

As a substitute, try making pizza at home, using homemade dough, low-sodium cheese, and your favorite vegetables as toppings.

PICKLES

Preserving any food requires salt. It stops the food from decaying and keeps it edible for longer.

The longer vegetables sit in canning and preserving liquids, the more sodium they pick up.

One small pickled cucumber contains 448 mg of sodium.
That said, reduced sodium options are available.

CANNED SOUPS

Canned soups are simple and easy to prepare, especially when you're crunched for time or not feeling well.

However, canned soups are high in sodium. Canned and packaged broths and stocks may contain similar amounts. This means they can elevate your blood pressure.

One can of tomato soup contains 1,110 mg of sodium, while a can of chicken and vegetable soup contains 2,140 mg.

Try choosing low or reduced-sodium soups instead, or make your soup at home from fresh ingredients.

CANNED TOMATO PRODUCTS

Most canned tomato sauces, pasta sauces, and tomato juices are high in sodium. This means they can raise your blood pressure, especially if you already have high blood pressure.

One serving (135 grams) of marinara sauce contains 566 mg of sodium. One cup of tomato juice contains 615 mg.

You can find low or reduced-sodium versions of most tomato products.

To lower your blood pressure, choose these alternatives or use fresh tomatoes, which are rich in an antioxidant called lycopene. Fresh vegetables have many heart-healthy benefits.

SUGAR

Sugar can increase your blood pressure in several ways.

Research indicates that sugar and especially sugar-sweetened drinks contribute to weight gain in adults and children. Being overweight or obese increases the chance of having high blood pressure.

Added sugar may also have a direct effect on increasing blood pressure, though more research is needed.

One 2019 study in females with high blood pressure reported that decreasing sugar by 2.3 teaspoons could result in an 8.4 mm Hg drop in systolic and a 3.7 mm Hg drop in diastolic blood pressure.

The AHA recommends the following daily added sugar limits:

6 Teaspoons, Or 25 Grams, For Females
9 Teaspoons, Or 36 Grams, For Males

PROCESSED FOODS WITH TRANS OR SATURATED FAT

To keep the heart healthy, it's best to reduce saturated fats and avoid trans fats. This is especially true for patients with high blood pressure

TRANS FATS are artificial fats that increase packaged foods' shelf life and stability.

However, eating them raises LDL (bad) cholesterol levels and lowers HDL (good) cholesterol levels, which can increase the risk of hypertension.

SATURATED FATS also increase the levels of LDL cholesterol in the blood.

Trans fats are especially harmful to your health and are linked to poor heart health, including an increased risk of:

- **HEART DISEASE**
- **STROKE**
- **TYPE 2 DIABETES**

Packaged, pre-prepared foods often contain trans fats and saturated fats, alongside high amounts of sugar, sodium, and low-fiber carbohydrates.

Saturated fats are mostly found in animal products, including:

- **FULL-FAT MILK AND CREAM**
- **BUTTER**
- **RED MEAT**
- **CHICKEN SKIN**

The AHA recommends reducing intake of both saturated and trans fats to help keep the heart healthy.

One way to reduce your saturated fat intake is to replace some animal foods with plant-based alternatives.

Many plant-based foods contain healthy monounsaturated and polyunsaturated fatty acids. Examples of plant-based foods include:

- **NUTS**
- **SEEDS**
- **OLIVE OIL**
- **AVOCADO**

According to our research in 2015, a full-fat dairy doesn't raise blood pressure.

ALCOHOL
Drinking too much alcohol can increase your blood pressure.

If you have high blood pressure, your doctor might recommend that you reduce the amount of alcohol you drink.

Following our research in 2017, a link between drinking less alcohol and lowering blood pressure among individuals who usually had more than two drinks each day.

In individuals who do not have hypertension, limiting alcohol intake may help reduce their risk of developing high blood pressure.

Alcohol can also prevent blood pressure medications that you may be taking from working effectively through drug interactions.

In addition, many alcoholic drinks are high in sugar and calories. Drinking alcohol can contribute to obesity and obesity, which can increase the risk of hypertension.

If you drink, limiting your alcohol intake to two drinks per day for males and one drink per day for females is recommended.

Does It Mean Individuals And Patients Trying To Avoid Or Lower High Blood Pressure Should Not Consume The Following Foods;

- BREAD AND ROLLS
- PIZZA
- SANDWICHES
- COLD CUTS AND CURED MEATS
- CANNED SOUP
- BURRITOS AND TACOS
- DELI MEAT

You can eat some of the above food as long as it is homemade with reduced fat ingredients and zero salts.

INTRODUCTION II

UNDERSTANDING BLOOD PRESSURE AND ITS IMPACT ON HEALTH

Blood pressure is a measurement of the force of blood against the walls of your arteries as your heart pumps it throughout your body. It is measured in millimeters of mercury (mmHg) and is recorded as two numbers: systolic pressure (top number) and diastolic pressure (bottom number). Systolic pressure is the pressure when your heart beats, while diastolic pressure is the pressure when your heart is resting between beats.

Blood pressure is an important indicator of overall health, and having high blood pressure (hypertension) can significantly increase your risk of developing serious health conditions such as heart disease, stroke, and kidney failure.
Understanding the impact of high blood pressure on your health is essential in preventing these conditions.

IMPACT OF HIGH BLOOD PRESSURE ON HEALTH

Heart Disease: High blood pressure is a major risk factor for heart disease. Over time, the excess pressure on the walls of your arteries can cause damage, making them stiff and narrow. This makes it harder for blood to flow through them, which can lead to a heart attack or heart failure.

STROKE: High blood pressure can also increase your risk of stroke. When the arteries in your brain become narrow or blocked, it can cause a stroke, which can result in permanent brain damage or even death.

KIDNEY DISEASE: The kidneys are responsible for filtering waste and excess fluid from your blood. High blood pressure can damage the blood vessels in your kidneys, making them less effective at filtering waste. Over time, this can lead to kidney disease, which can be life-threatening.

VISION LOSS: High blood pressure can damage the blood vessels in your eyes, leading to vision loss and even blindness.

UNDERSTANDING BLOOD PRESSURE READINGS

A blood pressure reading consists of two numbers: systolic pressure (top number) and diastolic pressure (bottom number). A normal blood pressure reading is typically around 120/80 mmHg.

If your blood pressure is consistently above 130/80 mmHg, you may be diagnosed with hypertension. If your blood pressure is above 180/120 mmHg, you may be experiencing a hypertensive crisis, which is a medical emergency.

CAUSES OF HIGH BLOOD PRESSURE

Several factors can contribute to high blood pressure, including:

- FAMILY HISTORY OF HIGH BLOOD PRESSURE

- UNHEALTHY DIET, PARTICULARLY ONE THAT IS HIGH IN SODIUM AND LOW IN POTASSIUM

- LACK OF PHYSICAL ACTIVITY

- BEING OVERWEIGHT OR OBESE

- SMOKING

- CHRONIC STRESS

- CERTAIN HEALTH CONDITIONS, SUCH AS SLEEP APNEA OR DIABETES

HEALTHY DIET TO MANAGE BLOOD PRESSURE

LOWER CHOLESTEROL LEVELS: A healthy diet that emphasizes whole foods and limits saturated and trans fats can help lower cholesterol levels. High cholesterol levels are a risk factor for heart disease, which can lead to high blood pressure.

REDUCED RISK OF STROKE AND HEART ATTACK: Eating a healthy diet helps to reduce your risk of stroke and heart attack by keeping your blood pressure under control.

IMPROVED ENERGY LEVELS:
Eating a healthy diet helps to provide
your body with the necessary nutrients it
needs to function properly. This will help
improve your energy levels and overall
well-being.

WEIGHT LOSS: Eating a healthy diet
can help you manage your weight and
reduce your risk of obesity and related
health conditions.

IMPROVED MENTAL HEALTH:
Eating a healthy diet can help to reduce
stress and anxiety levels, as well as
improve your mood.

**LOWER RISK OF DIABETES AND
OTHER
CHRONIC DISEASES**: Eating a
healthy diet can help to reduce your risk
of developing diabetes and other chronic

diseases, such as hypertension and high cholesterol.

TIPS FOR PLANNING A HEALTHY BLOOD PRESSURE DIET

FOODS THAT LOWER BLOOD:

LEAFY GREENS:
Leafy greens such as spinach, kale, and collard greens are rich in potassium, a mineral that can help lower blood pressure by counteracting the effects of sodium. They are also a good source of nitrates, which can improve blood flow and lower blood pressure.

BERRIES:

Berries such as blueberries and strawberries are rich in flavonoids, which are natural compounds that can help relax blood vessels and improve blood flow, thus reducing blood pressure.

BEETS:

Beets are rich in nitrates, which can help improve blood flow and lower blood pressure. Studies have shown that drinking beet juice can significantly lower blood pressure.

AVOCADO:

Avocado is a good source of potassium, a mineral that can help lower blood pressure by counteracting the effects of sodium. Avocado is also high in heart-healthy monounsaturated fats, which can help improve cholesterol levels.

GARLIC:
Garlic has been shown to have a mild blood pressure-lowering effect. It works by relaxing blood vessels and improving blood flow.

FISH:
Fatty fish such as salmon and mackerel are rich in omega-3 fatty acids, which can help reduce inflammation and lower blood pressure.

NUTS AND SEEDS:
Nuts and seeds are a good source of magnesium, a mineral that can help lower blood pressure by relaxing blood vessels.

WHOLE GRAINS:
Whole grains such as brown rice, quinoa, and oats are rich in fiber, which can help lower blood pressure by improving cholesterol levels and reducing inflammation.

LOW-FAT DAIRY:
Low-fat dairy products such as milk and yogurt are good sources of calcium and vitamin D, which can help lower blood pressure.

DARK CHOCOLATE:
Dark chocolate is rich in flavonoids, which can help improve blood flow and lower blood pressure.

POMEGRANATE:
Pomegranate juice is rich in antioxidants, which can help reduce inflammation and improve blood flow, thus lowering blood pressure.

WATERMELON:
Watermelon is rich in lycopene, a natural compound that can help relax blood vessels and lower blood pressure.

TOMATOES:
Tomatoes are rich in lycopene and other antioxidants, which can help improve blood flow and lower blood pressure.

TURMERIC:
Turmeric contains a compound called curcumin, which has been shown to have a mild blood pressure-lowering effect.

GREEN TEA:
Green tea is rich in catechins, natural compounds that can help relax blood vessels and improve blood flow, thus lowering blood pressure.

CITRUS FRUITS:
Citrus fruits such as oranges and grapefruits are rich in vitamin C, which can help improve blood flow and lower blood pressure.

LEGUMES:
Legumes such as beans, lentils, and chickpeas are rich in fiber and potassium, which can help lower blood pressure by relaxing blood vessels.

APPLE CIDER VINEGAR:
Apple cider vinegar has been shown to have a mild blood pressure-lowering effect. It works by reducing the activity of an enzyme that constricts blood vessels.

OLIVE OIL:
Olive oil is high in heart-healthy monounsaturated fats, which can help improve cholesterol levels and lower blood pressure.

CELERY:
Celery is rich in nitrates and other natural compounds that can help relax blood vessels and lower blood pressure.

NOTE: Incorporating these foods into your diet will help lower your blood pressure naturally.

CHAPTER 1: SAMPLE MENUS

MENU 1
Grilled Salmon with Orange-Thyme Glaze (30 minutes prep time)

INGREDIENTS:
- 4 (6-ounce) salmon filets
- 2 tablespoons extra-virgin olive oil
- 1/2 teaspoon sea salt
- 1/4 teaspoon freshly ground black pepper
- 1/4 cup freshly squeezed orange juice
- 2 tablespoons honey
- 1 teaspoon fresh thyme leaves

Cooking Method:
1. Preheat the grill to medium-high heat.

2. Brush the salmon filets with the olive oil and season with the salt and pepper.
3. Grill the salmon for 5 minutes per side, or until cooked through.
4. Meanwhile, in a small saucepan, combine the orange juice, honey, and thyme.
5. Bring to a boil over medium heat and cook for 5 minutes, stirring occasionally.
6. Remove from the heat and brush the glaze over the salmon.
7. Serve immediately.

MENU 2
Quinoa and Black Bean Salad (15 minutes prep time)

INGREDIENTS:
- -1 cup uncooked quinoa
- -2 cups cooked black beans
- -1/2 red onion, diced

- -1/2 red bell pepper, diced
- -1/2 cup freshly squeezed lime juice
- -3 tablespoons extra-virgin olive oil
- -1 teaspoon ground cumin
- -1/2 teaspoon sea salt
- -1/4 teaspoon freshly ground black pepper

Cooking Method:
1. Cook the quinoa according to package instructions.
2. In a large bowl, combine the cooked quinoa, black beans, onion, and bell pepper.
3. In a small bowl, whisk together the lime juice, olive oil, cumin, salt, and pepper.
4. Pour the dressing over the quinoa mixture and toss to combine.
5. Serve immediately or refrigerate for up to 3 days.

MENU 3
Roasted Vegetable and Chickpea Bowl (30 minutes prep time)

- INGREDIENTS:
- -1 sweet potato, diced
- -1 red bell pepper, seeded and diced
- -1 onion, diced
- -2 cloves garlic, minced
- -1 (15-ounce) can chickpeas, drained and rinsed
- -2 tablespoons extra-virgin olive oil
- -1 teaspoon ground cumin
- -1/2 teaspoon sea salt
- -1/4 teaspoon freshly ground black pepper
- -1/4 cup freshly squeezed lemon juice

Cooking Method:
1. Preheat the oven to 400°F.

2. In a large bowl, combine the sweet potato, bell pepper, onion, garlic, and chickpeas.

3. Drizzle with the olive oil and season with the cumin, salt, and pepper. Toss to combine.

4. Spread the vegetables in a single layer on a baking sheet.

5. Roast for 20 minutes, or until the vegetables are tender.

6. In a small bowl, whisk together the lemon juice and 1 tablespoon of water.

7.Drizzle the lemon mixture over the roasted vegetables and toss to combine.

8. Serve immediately.

MENU 4
Kale and Apple Salad (15 minutes prep time)

INGREDIENTS:

- -1 bunch kale, stems removed and leaves torn into bite-sized pieces
- -1 apple, cored and diced
- -1/4 cup freshly squeezed lemon juice
- -2 tablespoons extra-virgin olive oil
- -1/2 teaspoon sea salt
- -1/4 teaspoon freshly ground black pepper
- -1/4 cup slivered almonds

Cooking Method:

1. In a large bowl, combine the kale, apple, lemon juice, olive oil, salt, and pepper.

2. Massage the mixture with your hands until the kale starts to soften, about 2 minutes.

3. Add the slivered almonds and toss to combine.

4. Serve immediately.

MENU 5
Vegetable Stir-Fry (30 minutes prep time)

INGREDIENTS:
- -1 tablespoon sesame oil
- -1 onion, diced
- -2 cloves garlic, minced
- -1 red bell pepper, seeded and diced
- -1/2 cup sliced mushrooms
- -1/2 cup snow peas
- -1/2 cup diced carrots
- -1/4 cup low-sodium vegetable broth
- -1 tablespoon low-sodium soy sauce

Cooking Method:
1. Heat the sesame oil in a large skillet over medium heat.
2. Add the onion and garlic and cook for 2 minutes, stirring occasionally.

3. Add the bell pepper, mushrooms, snow peas, and carrots and cook for 5 minutes, stirring occasionally.
4. Add the vegetable broth and soy sauce and cook for an additional 5 minutes, stirring occasionally.
5. Serve immediately.

MENU 6
Baked Salmon with Honey-Mustard Glaze (30 minutes prep time)

INGREDIENTS:
- -4 (6-ounce) salmon filets
- -2 tablespoons extra-virgin olive oil
- -1/2 teaspoon sea salt
- -1/4 teaspoon freshly ground black pepper
- -2 tablespoons honey
- -2 tablespoons Dijon mustard

Cooking Method:
1. Preheat the oven to 375°F.
2. Brush the salmon filets with the olive oil and season with the salt and pepper.
3. Place the filets in a baking dish and bake for 15 minutes, or until cooked through.
4. Meanwhile, in a small bowl, whisk together the honey and mustard.
5. Brush the glaze over the cooked salmon.
6. Serve immediately.

MENU 7
Farro and Bean Salad (15 minutes prep time)

INGREDIENTS:
- -1 cup uncooked farro
- -2 cups cooked black beans
- -1/2 red onion, diced

- -1/2 red bell pepper, diced
- -3 tablespoons extra-virgin olive oil
- -1/4 cup freshly squeezed lemon juice
- -1 teaspoon dried oregano
- -1/2 teaspoon sea salt
- -1/4 teaspoon freshly ground black pepper

Cooking Method:
1. Cook the farro according to package instructions.
2. In a large bowl, combine the cooked farro, black beans, onion, and bell pepper.
3. In a small bowl, whisk together the olive oil, lemon juice, oregano, salt, and pepper.
4. Pour the dressing over the farro mixture and toss to combine.
5. Serve immediately or refrigerate for up to 3 days.

MENUS 8
Roasted Red Pepper and Tomato Soup (30 minutes prep time)

INGREDIENTS:
- -1 tablespoon extra-virgin olive oil
- -1 onion, diced
- -2 cloves garlic, minced
- -2 red bell peppers, seeded and diced
- -1 (28-ounce) can diced tomatoes
- -1 (14-ounce) can low-sodium vegetable broth
- -1/2 teaspoon dried oregano
- -1/2 teaspoon sea salt
- -1/4 teaspoon freshly ground black pepper

Cooking Method:

1. Heat the olive oil in a large pot over medium heat.
2. Add the onion and garlic and cook for 2 minutes, stirring occasionally.
3. Add the bell peppers, tomatoes, vegetable broth, oregano, salt, and pepper.
4. Bring to a boil, reduce the heat to low, and simmer for 20 minutes.
5. Using an immersion blender, blend the soup until smooth.
6. Serve immediately.

MENUS 9
Kale and Avocado Salad (15 minutes prep time)

- INGREDIENTS:
- -1 bunch kale, stems removed and leaves torn into bite-sized pieces
- -1 avocado, diced

- -1/4 cup freshly squeezed lemon juice
- -2 tablespoons extra-virgin olive oil
- -1/2 teaspoon sea salt
- -1/4 teaspoon freshly ground black pepper
- -1/4 cup slivered almonds

Cooking Method:
1. In a large bowl, combine the kale, avocado, lemon juice, olive oil, salt, and pepper.
2. Massage the mixture with your hands until the kale starts to soften, about 2 minutes.
3. Add the slivered almonds and toss to combine.
4. Serve immediately.

MENUS 10
Quinoa and Veggie Bowl (30 minutes prep time)

INGREDIENTS:
- -1 cup uncooked quinoa
- -1 tablespoon extra-virgin olive oil
- -1 onion, diced
- -2 cloves garlic, minced
- -1 red bell pepper, seeded and diced
- -1/2 cup sliced mushrooms
- -1/2 cup snow peas
- -1/2 cup diced carrots
- -1/4 cup low-sodium vegetable broth
- -1 tablespoon low-sodium soy sauce

Cooking Method:
1. Cook the quinoa according to package instructions.
2. Heat the olive oil in a large skillet over medium heat.

3. Add the onion and garlic and cook for 2 minutes,

RECIPES FOR BREAKFAST

1. Overnight Oats with Berries and Almonds

INGREDIENTS:
- ½ cup rolled oats,
- ½ cup almond milk,
- ½ cup fresh berries (such as blueberries or raspberries),
- 2 tablespoons slivered almonds

Cooking Method:
In a medium bowl, combine the oats, almond milk, and berries. Cover and refrigerate overnight. In the morning, stir in the almonds.
Prep Time: 5 minutes

Nutritional Value: Calories: 258, Fat: 10g, Carbohydrates: 33g, Protein: 9g

2. Avocado Toast with a Poached Egg

INGREDIENTS:
- 2 slices whole grain bread,
- 1 avocado, 2 eggs,
- 2 teaspoons white wine vinegar,
- 1 teaspoon olive oil

Cooking Method:
Toast the bread. Cut the avocado in half, remove the pit, and mash the flesh with a fork. Spread the avocado onto the toast slices.

Bring a pot of water to a boil over high heat and add the white wine vinegar. Reduce the heat to low and gently add the eggs, one at a time.

Cook for 3 minutes. Remove the eggs with a slotted spoon and place on top of the avocado toast. Drizzle with olive oil. Prep Time: 10 minutes

Nutritional Value: Calories: 397, Fat: 25g, Carbohydrates: 30g, Protein: 14g

3. Whole-Grain Pancakes with Blueberries

INGREDIENTS:
- 1 cup whole wheat flour,
- 1 teaspoon baking powder,
- 1 teaspoon baking soda,
- ¼ teaspoon ground cinnamon,
- ½ cup almond milk,
- 1 egg,
- 1 tablespoon olive oil,
- ½ cup fresh blueberries

Cooking Method:
In a medium bowl, combine the flour, baking powder, baking soda, and cinnamon.

In a separate bowl, whisk together the almond milk, egg, and olive oil. Add the wet ingredients to the dry ingredients and mix until just combined.
Gently fold in the blueberries.

Heat a lightly greased griddle or skillet over medium-high heat.

Drop ¼ cup of the batter onto the hot griddle and cook until the pancakes are lightly browned on each side, about 2 minutes per side.
Prep Time: 10 minutes

Nutritional Value: Calories: 304, Fat: 12g, Carbohydrates: 42g, Protein: 8g

4. Egg and Vegetable Scramble

INGREDIENTS:
- 2 eggs,
- 2 tablespoons almond milk,
- 1 small red pepper,
- ¼ cup diced mushrooms,
- 1 tablespoon olive oil

Cooking Method:
In a medium bowl, whisk together the eggs and almond milk. Set aside. In a large skillet over medium heat, heat the olive oil.

Add the red pepper and mushrooms and sauté for about 5 minutes, until the vegetables are softened. Pour the egg mixture into the skillet and stir until the eggs are cooked through.
Prep Time: 10 minutes

Nutritional Value: Calories: 151, Fat: 11g,
Carbohydrates: 5g, Protein: 9g

5. Greek Yogurt Bowl with Granola and Fruits

INGREDIENTS:
- 1 cup nonfat Greek yogurt,
- ¼ cup granola,
- 1 cup fresh fruit (such as strawberries, blueberries, or raspberries)
-

Cooking Method:
In a bowl, layer the Greek yogurt and granola. Top with the fresh fruit.
Prep Time: 5 minutes

Nutritional Value: Calories: 270, Fat: 5g,
Carbohydrates: 34g, Protein: 20g

6. Omelet with Spinach and Mushrooms Peanut Butter and Banana Toast:

INGREDIENTS:
- 2 slices of whole-grain bread,
- 2 tablespoons of natural peanut butter,
- 1 banana, sliced.

Optional:
1 tablespoon of honey, cinnamon

Cooking Method:
Toast the bread in a toaster or in a skillet. Spread peanut butter on one slice of bread and top it with banana slices. Place the other slice of bread on top.
Optional: Drizzle honey and sprinkle cinnamon on top.
Prep Time: 5 minutes

Nutritional Value: Calories- 350, Fat- 15 g, Carbs- 46 g, Protein- 11 g

7. Oatmeal with Nuts and Fruit:

INGREDIENTS:
- 1/2 cup of old-fashioned oats,
- 1 cup of hot water,
- 1/4 cup of chopped nuts (almonds, walnuts, etc.), 1/4 cup of diced fruits of your choice (apples, peaches, blueberries, etc.),
- 1 tablespoon of honey.

Optional: 1 tablespoon of chia seeds

Cooking Method: In a small saucepan, bring the water to a boil. Add the oats and stir until combined. Reduce the heat to medium-low and cook for 5 minutes, stirring occasionally. Add the nuts and diced fruits and stir until combined. Remove the oatmeal from the heat and stir in the honey. Optional: Stir in the chia seeds.

Prep Time: 10 minutes

Nutritional Value: Calories- 456, Fat- 24 g, Carbs- 47 g, Protein- 11 g

8.Steel-Cut Oats with Apples and Cinnamon:

INGREDIENTS:
- 1/2 cup of steel-cut oats,
- 1 cup of hot water,
- 1 apple, diced,
- 1 teaspoon of ground cinnamon.

Optional: 1 tablespoon of honey

Cooking Method:

In a small saucepan, bring the water to a boil. Add the oats and stir until combined. Reduce the heat to medium-low and cook for 10 minutes, stirring occasionally. Add the diced apples and cinnamon and stir until combined. Remove the oatmeal from the heat and stir in the honey.
Prep Time: 15 minutes

Nutritional Value: Calories- 385, Fat- 8 g, Carbs- 69 g, Protein- 12 g

9. Avocado and Egg Sandwich:

INGREDIENTS:
- 2 slices of whole-grain bread,
- 1/2 avocado, mashed,
- 2 eggs, cooked of your choice,
- 2 slices of tomato,
- 1 teaspoon of olive oil.

Optional: 1 tablespoon of hot sauce

Cooking Method:
Heat a skillet over medium heat and add the olive oil. Crack the eggs into the skillet and cook until desired doneness. Toast the bread in a toaster or in a skillet. Spread mashed avocado on one slice of bread and top it with tomato slices and cooked eggs. Place the other slice of bread on top. Optional: Drizzle hot sauce on top.
Prep Time: 10 minutes

Nutritional Value: Calories- 377, Fat- 23 g, Carbs- 28 g, Protein- 18 g

10. Veggie Omelet:

INGREDIENTS:
- 2 eggs,
- 2 tablespoons of water,
- 1/4 cup of diced vegetables of your choice (onion, bell pepper, spinach, etc.),
- 1 teaspoon of olive oil.

Optional: 1 tablespoon of grated cheese

Cooking Method:
In a small bowl, whisk together the eggs and water. Heat a skillet over medium heat and add the olive oil. Add the diced vegetables and sauté for 3 minutes. Pour the egg mixture into the skillet and cook until desired doneness. Optional: Sprinkle grated cheese on top.
Prep Time: 10 minutes

Nutritional Value: Calories- 150, Fat- 10 g, Carbs- 4 g, Protein- 13 g

11. Tofu Scramble with Mixed Vegetables:

INGREDIENTS:
- 1/2 block of extra-firm tofu, crumbled,
- 1/2 cup of diced vegetables of your choice (onion, bell pepper, mushrooms, etc.),
- 1 teaspoon of olive oil.

Optional: 1 tablespoon of nutritional yeast

Cooking Method:
Heat a skillet over medium heat and add the olive oil. Add the crumbled tofu and diced vegetables and sauté for 5 minutes. Optional: Sprinkle nutritional yeast on top.
Prep Time: 10 minutes

Nutritional Value: Calories- 180, Fat- 10 g, Carbs- 10 g, Protein- 14 g

12. Egg White Omelet with Spinach and Mushrooms:

INGREDIENTS:
- 3 egg whites,
- 1/4 cup of chopped spinach,
- 1/4 cup of sliced mushrooms,
- 1 teaspoon of olive oil.

Optional:
1 tablespoon of grated cheese

Cooking Method:
Heat a skillet over medium heat and add the olive oil. Add the egg whites, spinach, and mushrooms and cook until desired doneness.

Nutritional Value: Calories- 120, Fat- 5 g, Carbs- 4 g, Protein- 14 g

13. Muesli with Almond Milk

INGREDIENTS:
- - 2 cups rolled oats
- - 1 cup almond milk
- - ¼ cup dried cranberries
- - ¼ cup raisins
- - ¼ cup chopped walnuts
- - 2 tablespoons honey
- - 1 teaspoon ground cinnamon

Cooking Method:
1. Preheat the oven to 350°F.
2. Spread oats on a baking sheet and bake for 10 minutes, stirring once halfway through.

3. In a medium bowl, combine almond milk, cranberries, raisins, walnuts, honey and cinnamon.
4. Once the oats have finished baking, add to the bowl and mix to combine.
5. Serve warm or cold.
Prep Time: 15 minutes

Nutritional Value: Energy: 495 calories; Protein: 12g; Fat: 19g; Carbohydrates: 69g; Fiber: 10g; Sodium: 18mg.

14. Banana Smoothie Bowl

INGREDIENTS:
- - 2 ripe bananas
- - ½ cup almond milk
- - 1 tablespoon honey
- - 1 teaspoon ground cinnamon
- - 1 tablespoon chia seeds
- - 1 tablespoon coconut flakes

Cooking Method:
1. In a blender, combine bananas, almond milk, honey and cinnamon until smooth.
2. Pour into a bowl and top with chia seeds and coconut flakes.
Prep Time: 5 minutes

Nutritional Value: Energy: 241 calories; Protein: 3g; Fat: 6g; Carbohydrates: 44g; Fiber: 6g; Sodium: 33mg.

15. Chia Pudding with Nuts and Berries

INGREDIENTS:
- - 1 cup almond milk
- - ¼ cup chia seeds
- - 1 teaspoon honey

- - ½ cup mixed berries (fresh or frozen)
- - 2 tablespoons chopped nuts

Cooking Method:
1. In a medium bowl, combine almond milk, chia seeds and honey. Stir to combine.
2. Let mixture sit for at least 15 minutes, stirring occasionally.
3. Once thickened, top with berries and nuts.

Prep Time: 20 minutes

Nutritional Value: Energy: 275 calories; Protein: 6g; Fat: 14g; Carbohydrates: 33g; Fiber: 10g; Sodium: 58mg.

16. Apple and Walnut Muffins

INGREDIENTS:
- - 1 ½ cups whole wheat flour
- - 1 teaspoon baking powder
- - ½ teaspoon baking soda
- - 1 cup applesauce
- - ¼ cup honey
- - ¼ cup almond milk
- - 1 teaspoon vanilla extract
- - 1 teaspoon ground cinnamon
- - ½ cup chopped walnuts

Cooking Method:
1. Preheat the oven to 350°F.
2. In a medium bowl, combine flour, baking powder and baking soda.
3. In a separate bowl, combine applesauce, honey, almond milk, vanilla extract and cinnamon.
4. Add wet ingredients to dry ingredients and mix until just combined.
5. Fold in walnuts.

6. Divide batter into 12 muffin cups and bake for 25 minutes or until a toothpick inserted in the center comes out clean.
Prep Time: 30 minutes

Nutritional Value: Energy: 173 calories; Protein: 4g; Fat: 6g; Carbohydrates: 28g; Fiber: 3g; Sodium: 79 mg.

17. Whole-Grain Toast with Nut Butter and Banana

INGREDIENTS:
- - 2 slices whole-grain bread
- - 2 tablespoons nut butter
- - 1 banana, sliced

Cooking Method:
1. Toast bread in a toaster until golden brown.

2. Spread nut butter on each slice of toast.

3. Top with banana slices.

Prep Time: 5 minutes

Nutritional Value: Energy: 260 calories; Protein: 8g; Fat: 12g; Carbohydrates: 35g; Fiber: 6g; Sodium: 133 mg.

18. Veggie and Bean Burrito

INGREDIENTS:
- - 2 whole wheat tortillas
- - ½ cup cooked black beans
- - ½ cup cooked brown rice
- - ½ cup chopped bell pepper
- - ½ cup cooked corn
- - 2 tablespoons salsa
- - 1 tablespoon olive oil
- - ½ teaspoon ground cumin

- - 1 avocado, sliced

Cooking Method:
1. Heat olive oil in a large skillet over medium heat.
2. Add bell pepper and cook for 3-4 minutes.
3. Add beans, rice, corn and cumin and cook for 5 minutes.
4. Spread salsa on each tortilla.
5. Divide bean and rice mixture between tortillas and top with avocado slices.
6. Roll up burritos and serve.

Prep Time: 15 minutes

Nutritional Value: Energy: 564 calories; Protein: 14g; Fat: 28g; Carbohydrates: 70g; Fiber: 13g; Sodium: 903mg.

19. Quinoa Porridge with Apples

INGREDIENTS:
- • - 2 cups cooked quinoa
- • - 2 apples, cored and chopped
- • - 2 cups almond milk
- • - 2 tablespoons maple syrup
- • - 2 teaspoons ground cinnamon
- • - Pinch of ground nutmeg

Cooking Method:
1. In a medium saucepan, heat the quinoa, apples, almond milk, maple syrup, cinnamon, and nutmeg over medium heat.
2. Cook the mixture, stirring occasionally, until it is thickened, about 10 minutes.
3. Serve the porridge warm.

Prep Time: 20 minutes

Nutritional Value:
Calories: 366
Fat: 5g

Carbohydrates: 71g
Fiber: 10g
Protein: 11g

20. Chicken and Sweet Potato Hash

INGREDIENTS:
- - 2 tablespoons olive oil
- - 1 small onion, diced
- - 1 red bell pepper, diced
- - 2 cloves garlic, minced
- - 2 cups cooked, shredded chicken
- - 2 cups cooked sweet potatoes, diced
- - 1 teaspoon paprika
- - 1 teaspoon ground cumin
- - 1/4 teaspoon ground black pepper

Cooking Method:
1. In a large skillet, heat the olive oil over medium heat.

2. Add the onion and bell pepper and cook for 5 minutes, stirring occasionally.
3. Add the garlic, chicken, sweet potatoes, paprika, cumin, and black pepper. Cook for 10 minutes, stirring occasionally.
4. Serve the hash warm.

Prep Time: 20 minutes

Nutritional Value:
Calories: 400
Fat: 19g
Carbohydrates: 27g
Fiber: 6g
Protein: 30g

21. Chickpea and Vegetable Stew

INGREDIENTS:
- - 2 tablespoons olive oil
- - 1 onion, diced

- - 2 cloves garlic, minced
- - 1 bell pepper, diced
- - 2 carrots, diced
- - 2 celery stalks, diced
- - 2 cups cooked chickpeas
- - 1 teaspoon dried oregano
- - 1 teaspoon ground cumin
- - 1 teaspoon paprika
- - 1/4 teaspoon ground black pepper
- - 2 cups vegetable broth
- - 2 cups diced tomatoes
- - 2 cups cooked quinoa

Cooking Method:
1. In a large pot, heat the olive oil over medium heat.
2. Add the onion, garlic, bell pepper, carrots, and celery and cook for 5 minutes, stirring occasionally.
3. Add the chickpeas, oregano, cumin, paprika, and black pepper and cook for 5 minutes.

4. Add the vegetable broth and tomatoes and bring the mixture to a boil.
5. Reduce the heat to low and simmer for 10 minutes.
6. Add the quinoa and simmer for an additional 5 minutes.
7. Serve the stew warm.

Prep Time: 30 minutes

Nutritional Value:
Calories: 416
Fat: 11g
Carbohydrates: 62g
Fiber: 13g
Protein: 17g

22. Berry and Almond Milk Smoothie

INGREDIENTS:

- - 1 cup frozen berries
- - 1 banana, peeled and sliced
- - 2 cups almond milk
- - 2 tablespoons almond butter
- - 1 tablespoon honey

Cooking Method:
1. Place the berries, banana, almond milk, almond butter, and honey in a blender.
2. Blend the mixture on high until it is smooth.
3. Serve the smoothie immediately.

Prep Time: 10 minutes

Nutritional Value:
Calories: 368
Fat: 15g
Carbohydrates: 51g
Fiber: 7g
Protein: 10g

23. Oat and Nut Energy Balls

INGREDIENTS:

- - 1 cup rolled oats
- - 1/4 cup almonds, chopped
- - 1/4 cup walnuts, chopped
- - 1/4 cup peanut butter
- - 1/4 cup honey
- - 1/4 cup dark chocolate chips

Cooking Method:

1. Place the oats, almonds, walnuts, peanut butter, honey, and chocolate chips in a bowl.
2. Mix the INGREDIENTS until combined.
3. Form the mixture into 1-inch balls.
4. Serve the energy balls immediately or store them in an airtight container in the refrigerator.

Prep Time: 20 minutes

Nutritional Value:
Calories: 228
Fat: 12g
Carbohydrates: 28g
Fiber: 4g
Protein: 6g

24. Whole-Wheat Toast with Avocado

INGREDIENTS:
- - 2 slices whole-wheat bread
- - 1 ripe avocado, peeled, pitted, and mashed
- - 1/4 teaspoon ground black pepper

Cooking Method:
1. Toast the bread.
2. Spread the mashed avocado on the toast and sprinkle with black pepper.

3. Serve the toast immediately.

Prep Time: 10 minutes
Nutritional Value: Calories: 288, Fat:
16g, Carbohydrates: 32g, Fiber: 8g,
Protein: 7g

25. Kale and White Bean Frittata

INGREDIENTS:
- - 2 tablespoons olive oil
- - 1 small onion, diced
- - 2 cloves garlic, minced
- - 1 bunch kale, chopped
- - 2 cups cooked white beans
- - 8 eggs
- - 1/4 teaspoon ground black pepper

Cooking Method:
1. Preheat the oven to 350°F.

2. In a large oven-safe skillet, heat the olive oil over medium heat.
3. Add the onion and garlic and cook for 5 minutes, stirring occasionally.
4. Add the kale and cook for an additional 5 minutes.
5. Add the white beans and cook for an additional 2 minutes.
6. In a large bowl, whisk together the eggs and black pepper.
7. Pour the egg mixture into the skillet and cook for 5 minutes, stirring occasionally.
8. Place the skillet in the oven and bake for 10 minutes.
9. Serve the frittata warm.
Prep Time: 30 minutes

Nutritional Value:
Calories: 330
Fat: 18g
Carbohydrates: 24g
Fiber: 9g, Protein: 20g

BLOOD PRESSURE DOWN APPETIZER RECIPES

1. Hummus with Whole-Wheat Pita

INGREDIENTS:
- -1 can (15 ounces) chickpeas, drained and rinsed
- -2 tablespoons tahini
- -2 tablespoons freshly squeezed lemon juice
- -2 cloves garlic, minced
- -2 tablespoons extra-virgin olive oil
- -1/4 teaspoon ground cumin
- -Whole-wheat pita

Cooking Method:
1. In a food processor, combine the chickpeas, tahini, lemon juice, garlic, olive oil, and cumin.

2. Process until smooth and creamy, about 2 minutes, stopping to scrape down the sides of the bowl as needed.
3. Serve the hummus with whole-wheat pita.
Prep Time: 15 minutes

Nutritional Value (per serving):
Calories: 270, Fat: 12g, Sodium: 115mg, Carbohydrates: 32g, Fiber: 7g, Protein: 8g

2. Avocado Toast with Sun-Dried Tomatoes
INGREDIENTS:

- -1 ripe avocado, pitted and mashed
- -2 tablespoons sun-dried tomatoes, chopped
- -1 tablespoon freshly squeezed lemon juice

- -2 slices whole-wheat bread

Cooking Method:
1. In a small bowl, combine the mashed avocado, sun-dried tomatoes, and lemon juice.
2. Spread the avocado mixture on the whole-wheat bread slices.
3. Serve immediately.
Prep Time: 10 minutes

Nutritional Value (per serving):
Calories: 230, Fat: 15g, Sodium: 200mg, Carbohydrates: 21g, Fiber: 6g, Protein: 6g

3. Roasted Red Pepper and Feta Dip
INGREDIENTS:

- -1 red bell pepper

- -1/4 cup crumbled feta cheese
- -1/4 cup plain Greek yogurt
- -1 tablespoon extra-virgin olive oil
- -1 clove garlic, minced
- -Veggies and/or crackers, for serving

Cooking Method:
1. Preheat the oven to 425°F.
2. Place the bell pepper on a baking sheet and bake for 20 minutes, or until the skin is charred.
3. Remove the pepper from the oven and place it in a bowl. Cover the bowl with plastic wrap and let the pepper steam for 10 minutes.
4. Peel and discard the pepper's skin.
5. In a food processor, combine the roasted pepper, feta cheese, Greek yogurt, olive oil, and garlic. Process until smooth.
6. Serve the dip with veggies and/or crackers.

Prep Time: 30 minutes

Nutritional Value (per serving):
Calories: 90, Fat: 7g, Sodium: 220mg,
Carbohydrates: 4g, Fiber: 1g, Protein: 4g

4. Grilled Vegetable Platter with Balsamic Vinaigrette
INGREDIENTS:

- -1 red bell pepper, cut into strips
- -1 zucchini, cut into slices
- -1 yellow squash, cut into slices
- -1 red onion, cut into slices
- -1 tablespoon extra-virgin olive oil
- -1/4 cup balsamic vinegar
- -2 cloves garlic, minced

Cooking Method:
1. Preheat a grill or grill pan to medium-high heat.

2. Place the bell pepper, zucchini, yellow squash, and red onion on a baking sheet. Drizzle with the olive oil and toss to coat.
3. Place the vegetables on the grill and cook for 8-10 minutes, or until lightly charred and tender, flipping once halfway through.
4. In a small bowl, whisk together the balsamic vinegar, garlic, and remaining olive oil.
5. Serve the grilled vegetables with the balsamic vinaigrette.
Prep Time: 15 minutes

Nutritional Value (per serving):
Calories: 80, Fat: 4g, Sodium: 20mg, Carbohydrates: 8g, Fiber: 2g, Protein: 2g

5. Edamame and Bean Dip with Veggie Sticks
INGREDIENTS:

- -1 cup cooked edamame
- -1 can (15 ounces) black beans, drained and rinsed
- -1/4 cup freshly squeezed lime juice
- -1 tablespoon extra-virgin olive oil
- -1/4 teaspoon garlic powder
- -Veggie sticks, for serving

Cooking Method:
1. In a food processor, combine the edamame, black beans, lime juice, olive oil, and garlic powder. Process until smooth.
2. Serve the dip with veggie sticks.
Prep Time: 10 minutes

Nutritional Value (per serving):
Calories: 140, Fat: 5g, Sodium: 180mg, Carbohydrates: 16g, Fiber: 5g, Protein: 7g

6. Zucchini Fritters

INGREDIENTS:

- -2 cups grated zucchini
- -1/2 cup all-purpose flour
- -1 tablespoon minced fresh parsley
- -1/2 teaspoon garlic powder
- -1/4 teaspoon ground black pepper
- -1 large egg
- -1 tablespoon extra-virgin olive oil

Cooking Method:

1. Place the grated zucchini in a colander and sprinkle with salt. Let sit for 10 minutes, then squeeze out the excess liquid.
2. In a large bowl, combine the zucchini, flour, parsley, garlic powder, black pepper, and egg. Stir to combine.
3. Heat the olive oil in a large skillet over medium heat.

4. Drop spoonfuls of the zucchini mixture into the hot oil and cook for 3-4 minutes per side, or until golden brown.
5. Serve the fritters hot.
Prep Time: 20 minutes

Nutritional Value (per serving):
Calories: 120, Fat: 6g, Sodium: 40mg, Carbohydrates: 11g, Fiber: 2g, Protein: 5g

7. Guacamole with Baked Tortilla Chips
INGREDIENTS:

- -2 ripe avocados, pitted and mashed
- -1/4 cup diced onion
- -1/4 cup diced tomato
- -1 tablespoon freshly squeezed lime juice
- -1/4 teaspoon garlic powder
- -1/4 teaspoon ground cumin

- -Tortilla chips, for serving

Cooking Method:
1. In a medium bowl, combine the mashed avocados, onion, tomato, lime juice, garlic powder, and cumin.
2. Preheat the oven to 375°F.
3. Place the tortilla chips on a baking sheet and bake for 5 minutes, or until lightly golden.
4. Serve the guacamole with the baked tortilla chips.
Prep Time: 10 minutes

Nutritional Value (per serving):
Calories: 210, Fat: 15g, Sodium: 25mg, Carbohydrates: 19g, Fiber: 7g, Protein: 3g

8. Spinach Artichoke Dip
INGREDIENTS:

- -1 can (14 ounces) artichoke hearts, drained and chopped
- -1 package (10 ounces) frozen spinach, thawed and drained
- -1/2 cup plain Greek yogurt
- -1/2 cup grated Parmesan cheese
- -1/4 cup chopped scallions
- -1/4 teaspoon garlic powder
- -Veggies and/or crackers, for serving

Cooking Method:
1. Preheat the oven to 375°F.
2. In a large bowl, combine the artichoke hearts, spinach, Greek yogurt, Parmesan cheese, scallions, and garlic powder.
3. Transfer the mixture to an oven-safe baking dish.
4. Bake for 15 minutes, or until the dip is hot and bubbly.

5. Serve the dip hot with veggies and/or crackers.
Prep Time: 20 minutes

Nutritional Value (per serving):
Calories: 120, Fat: 7g, Sodium: 400mg, Carbohydrates: 8g, Fiber: 3g, Protein: 9g

9. Roasted Eggplant and Tomato Bruschetta
INGREDIENTS:

- -1 eggplant, cut into 1/2-inch cubes
- -1 tablespoon extra-virgin olive oil
- -1/4 teaspoon garlic powder
- -1/4 teaspoon ground black pepper
- -2 tomatoes, diced
- -2 tablespoons minced fresh basil
- -2 tablespoons freshly squeezed lemon juice
- -2 slices whole-wheat bread

Cooking Method:
1. Preheat the oven to 400°F.
2. Place the eggplant cubes on a baking sheet. Drizzle with the olive oil, garlic powder, and black pepper. Toss to coat.
3. Roast for 20 minutes, or until lightly golden.
4. In a medium bowl, combine the roasted eggplant, tomatoes, basil, and lemon juice.
5. Toast the whole-wheat bread slices.
6. Top the toasted bread slices with the eggplant-tomato mixture.
Prep Time: 25 minutes

Nutritional Value (per serving):
Calories: 170, Fat: 6g, Sodium: 140mg, Carbohydrates: 25g, Fiber: 7g, Protein: 6g

10. Asian-Style Chicken Skewers with Peanut Sauce
INGREDIENTS:

- -1 pound boneless, skinless chicken breasts, cut into 1-inch cubes
- -2 tablespoons low-sodium soy sauce
- -1 tablespoon honey
- -1 tablespoon freshly grated ginger
- -1 tablespoon toasted sesame oil
- -2 cloves garlic, minced
- -1/4 cup chunky peanut butter
- -1/4 cup warm water
- -2 tablespoons freshly squeezed lime juice

Cooking Method:
1. In a medium bowl, combine the chicken, soy sauce, honey, ginger, sesame oil, and garlic. Toss to coat.

2. Preheat a grill or grill pan to medium-high heat.

3. Thread the chicken onto skewers and grill for 10 minutes, or until cooked through, flipping once halfway through.

4. In a small bowl, whisk together the peanut butter, warm water, and lime juice.

5. Serve the chicken skewers with the peanut sauce.

Prep Time: 20 minutes

BLOOD PRESSURE LOWERING LUNCH RECIPES

1. Lentil and Vegetable Soup
INGREDIENTS:

- - 2 cups of lentils
- - 2 cloves of garlic, minced
- - 1 large onion, diced
- - 2 carrots, diced
- - 2 stalks of celery, diced
- - 2 potatoes, diced
- - 2 tablespoons of olive oil
- - 4 cups of vegetable broth
- - 1 teaspoon of dried oregano
- - 1 teaspoon of dried thyme
- - Salt and pepper to taste

Cooking Method:

1. Heat the olive oil in a large pot over medium heat.
2. Add the garlic, onion, carrots, and celery to the pot and sauté until the vegetables are softened, about 5 minutes.
3. Add the potatoes, lentils, and vegetable broth to the pot and bring to a boil.
4. Reduce the heat to low and simmer for 30 minutes, stirring occasionally.
5. Add the oregano, thyme, salt, and pepper and simmer for an additional 10 minutes.
6. Serve the soup hot.

Nutritional Value:
- Calories: 370
- Protein: 18g
- Fat: 9g
- Carbohydrates: 56g
- Fiber: 17g
Prep Time: 15 minutes
Cook Time: 45 minutes

2. Quinoa and Black Bean Burrito

INGREDIENTS:

- - 1 cup of quinoa, cooked
- - 1 can of black beans, rinsed and drained
- - 1 teaspoon of olive oil
- - 1 red bell pepper, diced
- - 1 onion, diced
- - 1 jalapeño, diced
- - 2 cloves of garlic, minced
- - 2 teaspoons of chili powder
- - 2 teaspoons of ground cumin
- - 2 tablespoons of fresh cilantro, chopped
- - 4 large tortillas
- - 2 avocados, sliced
- - 2 limes, cut into wedges
- - Salt and pepper to taste

Cooking Method:

1. Heat the olive oil in a large skillet over medium heat.

2. Add the onion, bell pepper, jalapeño, and garlic to the pan and sauté until the vegetables are softened, about 5 minutes.

3. Add the black beans, chili powder, cumin, salt, and pepper to the pan and cook for an additional 5 minutes.

4. Remove the pan from the heat and add the quinoa and cilantro to the pan. Stir to combine.

5. Place the tortillas on a work surface and divide the quinoa and black bean mixture evenly among them.
6. Top each tortilla with avocado slices and a squeeze of lime juice.
7. Roll the tortillas up and serve.

Nutritional Value:

- Calories: 498
- Protein: 16g
- Fat: 17g
- Carbohydrates: 74g
- Fiber: 15g
Prep Time: 15 minutes
Cook Time: 10 minutes

3. Broccoli and Kale Stir-Fry
INGREDIENTS:
- - 1 tablespoon of sesame oil
- - 1 onion, diced
- - 2 cloves of garlic, minced
- - 2 cups of broccoli florets
- - 2 cups of kale, chopped
- - 2 tablespoons of soy sauce
- - 2 tablespoons of rice vinegar
- - Salt and pepper to taste

Cooking Method:

1. Heat the sesame oil in a large skillet over medium heat.

2. Add the onion and garlic to the pan and sauté until the vegetables are softened, about 5 minutes.

3. Add the broccoli and kale to the pan and cook for an additional 5 minutes, stirring occasionally.

4. Add the soy sauce, rice vinegar, salt, and pepper and cook for an additional 5 minutes.
5. Serve the stir-fry hot.

Nutritional Value:
- Calories: 126
- Protein: 5g
- Fat: 6g
- Carbohydrates: 17g
- Fiber: 5g

Prep Time: 10 minutes
Cook Time: 10 minutes

4. Baked Sweet Potato with Steamed
Vegetables
INGREDIENTS:
- • - 2 sweet potatoes, peeled and cut
  into cubes
- • - 2 tablespoons of olive oil
- • - 1 cup of broccoli florets
- • - 1 cup of cauliflower florets
- • - 1 cup of carrots, sliced
- • - 1 teaspoon of dried thyme
- • - Salt and pepper to taste

Cooking Method:
1. Preheat the oven to 400°F.

2. Place the sweet potato cubes on a
baking sheet and toss with the olive oil.

3. Bake for 25 minutes, stirring halfway through.

4. While the sweet potatoes are baking, steam the broccoli, cauliflower, and carrots until they are tender, about 10 minutes.

5. Remove the sweet potatoes from the oven and toss with the thyme, salt, and pepper.

6. Serve the sweet potatoes with the steamed vegetables.

Nutritional Value:
- Calories: 298
- Protein: 6g
- Fat: 12g
- Carbohydrates: 44g
- Fiber: 9g
Prep Time: 10 minutes
Cook Time: 35 minutes

5. Avocado and Black Bean Wrap

INGREDIENTS:

- - 2 tablespoons of olive oil
- - 1 onion, diced
- - 2 cloves of garlic, minced
- - 1 can of black beans, rinsed and drained
- - 1 teaspoon of chili powder
- - 2 avocados, mashed
- - 4 large tortillas
- - 1 cup of spinach leaves
- - Salt and pepper to taste

Cooking Method:

1. Heat the olive oil in a large skillet over medium heat.

2. Add the onion and garlic to the pan and sauté until the vegetables are softened, about 5 minutes.

3. Add the black beans, chili powder, salt, and pepper to the pan and cook for an additional 5 minutes.

4. Place the tortillas on a work surface and spread each one with the mashed avocado.

5. Top the avocado with the black bean mixture and spinach leaves.

6. Roll the tortillas up and serve.

Nutritional Value:
- Calories: 498
- Protein: 15g
- Fat: 17g
- Carbohydrates: 72g
- Fiber: 15g
Prep Time: 10 minutes
Cook Time: 10 minutes

6. Hummus and Roasted Vegetable Wrap

INGREDIENTS:

- - 1 tablespoon of olive oil
- - 1 red bell pepper, cut into strips
- - 1 zucchini, cut into strips
- - 1 onion, cut into strips
- - 1 teaspoon of dried oregano
- - 4 large tortillas
- - 1 cup of hummus
- - 1 cup of spinach leaves
- - Salt and pepper to taste

Cooking Method:

1. Preheat the oven to 425°F.

2. Place the bell pepper, zucchini, and onion on a baking sheet and toss with the olive oil and oregano.

3. Bake for 20 minutes, stirring halfway through.

4. Place the tortillas on a work surface and spread each one with the hummus.
5. Top the hummus with the roasted vegetables and spinach leaves.

6. Roll the tortillas up and serve.

Nutritional Value:
- Calories: 472
- Protein: 11g
- Fat: 17g
- Carbohydrates: 70g
- Fiber: 10g
Prep Time: 10 minutes
Cook Time: 20 minutes

7. Roasted Vegetable and Quinoa Salad
INGREDIENTS:
- - 2 tablespoons of olive oil

- - 1 red bell pepper, cut into strips
- - 1 zucchini, cut into strips
- - 1 onion, cut into strips
- - 1 teaspoon of dried oregano
- - 2 cups of cooked quinoa
- - 2 tablespoons of fresh parsley, chopped
- - Salt and pepper to taste

Cooking Method:
1. Preheat the oven to 425°F.
2. Place the bell pepper, zucchini, and onion on a baking sheet and toss with the olive oil and oregano.
3. Bake for 20 minutes, stirring halfway through.
4. Place the quinoa in a large bowl and add the roasted vegetables.
5. Add the parsley, salt, and pepper and stir to combine.
6. Serve the salad at room temperature or chilled.

Nutritional Value:
- Calories: 296
- Protein: 9g
- Fat: 9g
- Carbohydrates: 43g
- Fiber: 7g
Prep Time: 10 minutes
Cook Time: 20 minutes

8. Whole Wheat Pasta with Tomato Sauce

INGREDIENTS:

- - 2 tablespoons of olive oil
- - 1 onion, diced
- - 2 cloves of garlic, minced
- - 1 can of crushed tomatoes
- - 1 teaspoon of dried oregano
- - 1 teaspoon of dried basil
- - 12 ounces of whole wheat pasta
- - Salt and pepper to taste

Cooking Method:

1. Heat the olive oil in a large pot over medium heat.

2. Add the onion and garlic to the pot and sauté until the vegetables are softened, about 5 minutes.

3. Add the crushed tomatoes, oregano, basil, salt, and pepper and bring to a boil.

4. Reduce the heat to low and simmer for 15 minutes, stirring occasionally.

5. Meanwhile, cook the pasta according to the package instructions.

6. Drain the pasta and add it to the pot with the tomato sauce.

7. Stir to combine and serve.

Nutritional Value:
- Calories: 477

- Protein: 16g
- Fat: 8g
- Carbohydrates: 81g
- Fiber: 10g
Prep Time: 10 minutes
Cook Time: 30 minutes

9. Grilled Vegetable and Hummus Sandwich

INGREDIENTS:

- - 2 tablespoons of olive oil
- - 1 red bell pepper, cut into strips
- - 1 zucchini, cut into strips
- - 1 onion, cut into strips
- - 1 teaspoon of dried oregano
- - 4 slices of whole wheat bread
- - 1 cup of hummus
- - Salt and pepper to taste

Cooking Method:
1. Heat the olive oil in a large skillet over medium heat.

2. Add the bell pepper, zucchini, and onion to the pan and toss with the oregano, salt, and pepper.

3. Cook for 10 minutes, stirring occasionally.

4. Place the bread slices on a work surface and spread each one with the hummus.

5. Top the hummus with the grilled vegetables.

6. Place the sandwiches in the skillet and cook until the bread is toasted, about 5 minutes per side.

7. Serve the sandwiches hot.

Nutritional Value:
- Calories: 486
- Protein: 12g

- Fat: 19g
- Carbohydrates: 66g
- Fiber: 11g
Prep Time: 10 minutes
Cook Time: 20 minutes

10. Baked Salmon with Roasted Vegetables

INGREDIENTS:
- 6 ounces of salmon
- 1 cup of chopped bell peppers
- 1 cup of chopped carrots
- 1/2 cup of chopped onions
- 1/4 cup of olive oil
- Salt and pepper to taste

Cooking Method:
1. Preheat the oven to 375°F.

2. Place the chopped bell peppers, carrots and onions on a baking sheet.

3. Drizzle with the olive oil and season with salt and pepper.

4. Place the salmon on top of the vegetables.

5. Bake in the preheated oven for 20 minutes or until the salmon is cooked through.

Nutritional Value:
Calories: 260 kcal
Carbs: 7 g
Protein: 19 g
Fat: 16 g
Prep Time: 10 minutes

11. Chickpea and Vegetable Curry
INGREDIENTS:
- 1 tablespoon of olive oil
- 1 cup of chopped onions

- 1 cup of chopped carrots
- 1 cup of chopped bell peppers
- 1 cup of cooked chickpeas
- 1/2 teaspoon of ground cumin
- 1/2 teaspoon of ground coriander
- 1/4 teaspoon of ground turmeric
- 1/4 teaspoon of chili powder
- 1/2 teaspoon of salt
- 1/4 teaspoon of black pepper
- 1 cup of coconut milk

Cooking Method:
1. Heat the olive oil in a large pot over medium-high heat.

2. Add the onions, carrots and bell peppers and cook until the vegetables are softened, about 5 minutes.

3. Add the cooked chickpeas and all of the spices and stir to combine.

4. Pour in the coconut milk and bring the mixture to a boil.

5. Reduce the heat to low and simmer for 15 minutes, stirring occasionally.

Nutritional Value:
Calories: 252 kcal
Carbs: 21 g
Protein: 8 g
Fat: 15 g
Prep Time: 15 minutes

12. Bean and Vegetable Burrito Bowl
INGREDIENTS:
- 1 tablespoon of olive oil
- 1 cup of chopped onions

- 1 cup of chopped bell peppers
- 1 cup of cooked black beans
- 1/2 teaspoon of ground cumin
- 1/2 teaspoon of chili powder
- 1/4 teaspoon of salt
- 1/4 teaspoon of black pepper
- 1 cup of cooked brown rice
- 1/2 cup of shredded cheese
- 1/4 cup of chopped cilantro
- 1/4 cup of sour cream

Cooking Method:
1. Heat the olive oil in a large skillet over medium heat.

2. Add the onions and bell peppers and cook until softened, about 5 minutes.

3. Add the cooked black beans, cumin, chili powder, salt and pepper and cook for another 5 minutes.

4. Place the cooked brown rice in a serving bowl.

5. Top with the cooked bean and vegetable mixture, cheese, cilantro and sour cream.

Nutritional Value:
Calories: 419 kcal
Carbs: 46 g
Protein: 15 g
Fat: 19 g
Prep Time: 15 minutes

13. Egg and Vegetable Frittata
INGREDIENTS:
- 1 tablespoon of olive oil
- 1 cup of chopped onions
- 1 cup of chopped bell peppers
- 1/2 cup of chopped mushrooms
- 6 eggs

- 1/4 teaspoon of salt
- 1/4 teaspoon of black pepper
- 1/4 cup of grated cheese

Cooking Method:
1. Preheat the oven to 375°F.

2. Heat the olive oil in a large skillet over medium heat.

3. Add the onions, bell peppers and mushrooms and cook until softened, about 5 minutes.

4. In a large bowl, whisk together the eggs, salt and pepper.

5. Pour the egg mixture into the skillet and cook until the eggs are just set, about 3 minutes.

6. Sprinkle with the grated cheese and transfer the skillet to the preheated oven.

7. Bake for 10 minutes or until the eggs are completely set.

Nutritional Value:
Calories: 217 kcal
Carbs: 4 g
Protein: 15 g
Fat: 15 g
Prep Time: 10 minutes

14. Roasted Eggplant and Quinoa Salad

INGREDIENTS:

- 1 tablespoon of olive oil
- 1 eggplant, cut into cubes
- 1/2 teaspoon of salt
- 1/4 teaspoon of black pepper
- 1 cup of cooked quinoa
- 1/4 cup of chopped parsley
- 1/4 cup of crumbled feta cheese
- 1/4 cup of chopped olives

- 2 tablespoons of olive oil
- 1 tablespoon of lemon juice

Cooking Method:
1. Preheat the oven to 400°F.

2. Place the cubed eggplant on a baking sheet and drizzle with the olive oil.

3. Sprinkle with the salt and pepper and roast in the preheated oven for 25 minutes.

4. In a large bowl, combine the cooked quinoa, roasted eggplant, parsley, feta cheese and olives.

5. Drizzle with the olive oil and lemon juice and toss to combine.

Nutritional Value:
Calories: 297 kcal
Carbs: 24 g

Protein: 8 g

Fat: 17 g

Prep Time: 10 minutes

15. Avocado and Roasted Vegetable Wrap

INGREDIENTS:

- 1 tablespoon of olive oil
- 1 cup of chopped bell peppers
- 1 cup of chopped carrots
- 1/2 cup of chopped onions
- 1/4 teaspoon of salt
- 1/4 teaspoon of black pepper
- 1 avocado, mashed
- 4 tortillas
- 1/4 cup of shredded cheese

Cooking Method:

1. Preheat the oven to 375°F.

2. Place the chopped bell peppers, carrots and onions on a baking sheet.

3. Drizzle with the olive oil and season with salt and pepper.

4. Roast in the preheated oven for 20 minutes.

5. In a small bowl, mash the avocado.

6. Spread the mashed avocado onto the tortillas.

7. Top with the roasted vegetables and shredded cheese.

8. Roll up the tortillas and enjoy.

Nutritional Value:
Calories: 281 kcal
Carbs: 23 g
Protein: 8 g

Fat: 17 g
Prep Time: 15 minutes

16. Turkey and Bean Chili
INGREDIENTS:

- 1 tablespoon of olive oil
- 1 pound of ground turkey
- 1 cup of chopped onions
- 1 cup of chopped bell peppers
- 1 teaspoon of ground cumin
- 1 teaspoon of chili powder
- 1/2 teaspoon of salt
- 1/4 teaspoon of black pepper
- 1 can of black beans, drained and rinsed
- 1 can of diced tomatoes
- 1/4 cup of chopped cilantro

Cooking Method:
1. Heat the olive oil in a large pot over medium-high heat.

2. Add the ground turkey and cook until it is browned, about 5 minutes.

3. Add the onions and bell peppers and cook until softened, about 5 minutes.

4. Add the cumin, chili powder, salt and pepper and stir to combine.

5. Add the black beans, tomatoes and 1 cup of water and bring the mixture to a boil.

6. Reduce the heat to low and simmer for 20 minutes, stirring occasionally.

7. Stir in the cilantro and serve.

Nutritional Value:
Calories: 314 kcal
Carbs: 21 g
Protein: 25 g
Fat: 14 g

Prep Time: 15 minutes

17. Greek Salad with Feta Cheese

INGREDIENTS:

- 2 cups of romaine lettuce, chopped
- 1/2 cup of chopped cucumber
- 1/2 cup of cherry tomatoes, halved
- 1/4 cup of sliced red onion
- 1/4 cup of pitted Kalamata olives
- 1/4 cup of crumbled feta cheese
- 1/4 cup of olive oil
- 1 tablespoon of lemon juice
- 1/2 teaspoon of oregano
- Salt and pepper to taste

Cooking Method:

1. In a large bowl, combine the romaine lettuce, cucumber, cherry tomatoes, red onion and Kalamata olives.

2. In a small bowl, whisk together the olive oil, lemon juice, oregano, salt and pepper.

3. Pour the dressing over the salad and toss to combine.

4. Sprinkle with the feta cheese and serve.

Nutritional Value:
Calories: 272 kcal
Carbs: 8 g
Protein: 6 g
Fat: 24 g
Prep Time: 10 minutes

18. Veggie Wrap with Hummus

INGREDIENTS:

- 1/4 cup of hummus
- 2 tortillas
- 1/2 cup of shredded lettuce
- 1/2 cup of chopped bell peppers
- 1/2 cup of chopped cucumber
- 1/4 cup of shredded carrots
- 1/4 cup of chopped walnuts

Cooking Method:

1. Spread the hummus onto the tortillas.

2. Place the lettuce, bell peppers, cucumber, carrots and walnuts on top of the hummus.

3. Roll up the tortillas and enjoy.

Nutritional Value:
Calories: 267 kcal
Carbs: 28 g

Protein: 8 g
Fat: 14 g
Prep Time: 10 minutes

19. Zucchini Noodles with Pesto
INGREDIENTS:
- 3-4 medium zucchini, spiraled into noodles
- 1/4 cup pesto
- 1/4 cup pine nuts
- 1/4 cup grated parmesan cheese
- Salt and pepper to taste

Cooking Method:
1. Preheat the oven to 400°F.

2. Place the zucchini noodles onto a baking sheet and bake for 10 minutes.

3. Remove from the oven and place the noodles into a large bowl.

4. Drizzle with the pesto and mix to combine.

5. Top with pine nuts, parmesan cheese, salt and pepper and mix again.

6. Serve warm.

Nutritional Value:
Calories: 175, Fat: 13g, Carbohydrates: 10g, Protein: 7g
Prep Time: 10 minutes

20. Cauliflower and Chickpea Salad
INGREDIENTS:
- 1 head cauliflower, cut into florets
- 1 can chickpeas, rinsed and drained
- 1/4 cup extra-virgin olive oil
- 2 cloves garlic, minced
- 1/2 teaspoon ground cumin
- 1/2 teaspoon paprika
- 1/2 teaspoon ground coriander

- 1/4 teaspoon cayenne pepper

Cooking Method:
1. Preheat the oven to 400°F.

2. Place the cauliflower and chickpeas onto a baking sheet and mix with the olive oil, garlic, cumin, paprika, coriander, cayenne pepper, salt and pepper.

3. Bake for 20 minutes, stirring halfway through.

4. Remove from the oven and let cool.

5. Serve chilled or at room temperature.

Nutritional Value:
Calories: 186, Fat: 11g, Carbohydrates: 17g, Protein: 6g
Prep Time: 25 minutes

21. Lentil and Vegetable Wraps
INGREDIENTS:
- 1 cup cooked lentils
- 1/4 cup diced red onion
- 1/4 cup diced bell pepper
- 1/4 cup diced cucumber
- 1/4 cup diced tomatoes
- 1/4 cup crumbled feta cheese
- 1/4 cup chopped parsley
- 2 tablespoons olive oil
- 2 tablespoons lemon juice
- Salt and pepper to taste
- 4 wraps

Cooking Method:
1. In a large bowl, combine the lentils, red onion, bell pepper, cucumber, tomatoes, feta cheese, parsley, olive oil, lemon juice, salt and pepper.

2. Mix until combined.

3. Divide the mixture among the wraps and roll up.

4. Serve chilled or at room temperature.

Nutritional Value:
Calories: 297, Fat: 12g, Carbohydrates: 34g, Protein: 11g
Prep Time: 15 minutes

22. Cold Quinoa and Vegetable Salad
INGREDIENTS:
- 1 cup cooked quinoa
- 1/2 cup diced red pepper
- 1/2 cup diced cucumber
- 1/2 cup diced tomatoes
- 1/4 cup crumbled feta cheese
- 1/4 cup chopped parsley
- 2 tablespoons olive oil
- 2 tablespoons lemon juice

- Salt and pepper to taste

Cooking Method:
1. In a large bowl, combine the quinoa, red pepper, cucumber, tomatoes, feta cheese, parsley, olive oil, lemon juice, salt and pepper.

2. Mix until combined.

3. Serve chilled or at room temperature.

Nutritional Value:
Calories: 199, Fat: 9g, Carbohydrates: 21g, Protein: 6g
Prep Time: 10 minutes

23. Spinach and Feta Omelet
INGREDIENTS:
- 2 eggs
- 2 tablespoons water
- 1/4 cup chopped spinach

- 2 tablespoons crumbled feta cheese
- Salt and pepper to taste
- 1 teaspoon olive oil

Cooking Method:

1. In a medium bowl, whisk together the eggs and water until combined.

2. Add the spinach, feta cheese, salt and pepper and mix to combine.

3. Heat the olive oil in a medium skillet over medium heat.

4. Pour in the egg mixture and cook for 2-3 minutes, until the edges begin to set.

5. Flip the omelet and cook for another 2 minutes, until cooked through.

6. Serve warm.

Nutritional Value:

Calories: 159, Fat: 11g, Carbohydrates: 2g, Protein: 11g
Prep Time: 10 minutes

24. Grilled Vegetable and Brown Rice Bowl

INGREDIENTS:
- 1 cup cooked brown rice
- 1 red bell pepper, cut into strips
- 1 zucchini, cut into slices
- 1 yellow squash, cut into slices
- 1 onion, cut into wedges
- 2 tablespoons olive oil
- Salt and pepper to taste

Cooking Method:

1. Preheat a grill to medium-high heat.

2. Place the bell pepper, zucchini, yellow squash and onion onto a baking sheet.

3. Drizzle with the olive oil, salt and pepper and toss to combine.

4. Place the vegetables onto the grill and cook for 10 minutes, or until lightly charred and tender.

5. Serve the vegetables over the cooked brown rice.

Nutritional Value:
Calories: 281, Fat: 9g, Carbohydrates: 39g, Protein: 7g
Prep Time: 15 minutes

25. Baked Tofu with Steamed Vegetables
INGREDIENTS:
- 1 block tofu, cut into cubes
- 1 cup broccoli florets
- 1 cup cauliflower florets
- 1 cup sliced bell pepper

- 2 tablespoons olive oil
- 2 tablespoons soy sauce
- 2 cloves garlic, minced
- Salt and pepper to taste

Cooking Method:
1. Preheat the oven to 400°F.

2. Place the tofu cubes onto a baking sheet and drizzle with the olive oil, soy sauce, garlic, salt and pepper.

3. Bake for 15 minutes.

4. Meanwhile, place the broccoli, cauliflower and bell pepper into a steamer basket and steam for 5-7 minutes, or until tender.

5. Serve the tofu and vegetables together.

Nutritional Value:

Calories: 313, Fat: 16g, Carbohydrates: 18g, Protein: 23g
Prep Time: 25 minutes

26. White Bean and Roasted Pepper Salad

INGREDIENTS:

- 1 can white beans, rinsed and drained
- 1 red bell pepper, cut into strips
- 1 yellow bell pepper, cut into strips
- 2 cloves garlic, minced
- 1 tablespoon olive oil
- 2 tablespoons red wine vinegar
- 1 tablespoon chopped parsley
- Salt and pepper to taste

Cooking Method:

1. Preheat the oven to 400°F.

2. Place the bell pepper strips on a baking sheet.

3. Drizzle with the olive oil and bake for 20 minutes, or until lightly charred.

4. Remove from the oven and let cool.

5. In a large bowl, combine the white beans, bell peppers, garlic, red wine vinegar, parsley, salt and pepper.

6. Mix until combined.

7. Serve chilled or at room temperature.

Nutritional Value:
Calories: 174, Fat: 5g, Carbohydrates: 25g, Protein: 7g
Prep Time: 25 minutes

27. Grilled Vegetable Sandwich with Hummus
INGREDIENTS:
- 2 slices whole wheat bread

- 2 tablespoons hummus
- 1/4 cup grilled vegetables (such as bell pepper, zucchini, onion, etc.)
- 1/4 cup crumbled feta cheese

Cooking Method:
1. Preheat a grill to medium-high heat.

2. Grill the vegetables until lightly charred and tender.

3. Spread the hummus onto the bread slices.

4. Top with the grilled vegetables, feta cheese, salt and pepper.

5. Grill the sandwich until the bread is lightly toasted, about 2-3 minutes per side.

6. Serve warm.

Nutritional Value:
Calories: 218, Fat: 10g, Carbohydrates:
23g, Protein: 10g
Prep Time: 10 minutes

28. Roasted Cauliflower and Quinoa Bowl

INGREDIENTS:
- 1 head cauliflower, cut into florets
- 1 cup cooked quinoa
- 2 tablespoons olive oil
- 2 cloves garlic, minced
- 1/2 teaspoon ground cumin
- 1/2 teaspoon paprika
- 1/2 teaspoon ground coriander
- 1/4 teaspoon cayenne pepper
- Salt and pepper to taste

Cooking Method:
1. Preheat the oven to 400°F.

2. Place the cauliflower onto a baking sheet and mix with the olive oil, garlic, cumin, paprika, coriander, cayenne pepper, salt and pepper.

3. Bake for 20 minutes, stirring halfway through.

4. Remove from the oven and let cool.

5. Serve the cauliflower over the cooked quinoa.

Nutritional Value:
Calories: 229, Fat: 11g, Carbohydrates: 25g, Protein: 8g
Prep Time: 25 minutes

29. Lentil and Vegetable Stew
INGREDIENTS:
- 1 cup cooked lentils
- 1 cup diced tomatoes

- 1/2 cup diced carrots
- 1/2 cup diced potatoes
- 1/2 cup diced celery
- 1 onion, diced
- 2 cloves garlic, minced
- 2 tablespoons olive oil
- 1 teaspoon dried oregano
- 1 teaspoon dried thyme

Cooking Method:
1. Heat the olive oil in a large pot over medium heat.

2. Add the onion and garlic and cook until softened, about 5 minutes.

3. Add the tomatoes, carrots, potatoes, celery, oregano, thyme, salt and pepper.

4. Bring to a simmer and cook for 15 minutes, or until the vegetables are tender.

5. Add the cooked lentils and cook for another 5 minutes.

6. Serve warm.

Nutritional Value:
Calories: 241, Fat: 7g, Carbohydrates: 33g, Protein: 12g
Prep Time: 25 minutes

CHAPTER 2: BLOOD PRESSURE DOWN DINNER RECIPES

Salmon With Roasted Vegetables

Prep Time: 15 minutes | Cook Time: 30 minutes | Total Time: 45 minutes

INGREDIENTS:
- - 4 4-ounce salmon filets
- - 1 red bell pepper, diced
- - 1 yellow bell pepper, diced
- - 1 zucchini, diced
- - 1 yellow squash, diced
- - 2 tablespoons olive oil
- - Salt and pepper, to taste

Cooking method
1. Preheat the oven to 400°F.

2. Place the diced vegetables on a baking sheet and drizzle with olive oil, salt and pepper.
3. Roast for 15 minutes.
4. Place the salmon filets on a separate baking sheet and drizzle with olive oil, salt and pepper.
5. Roast for 15 minutes.
6. Serve the salmon and roasted vegetables together.

Baked Cod With Lemon And Capers
Prep Time: 10 minutes | Cook Time: 20 minutes | Total Time: 30 minutes

INGREDIENTS:
- - 4 4-ounce cod filets
- - 2 tablespoons olive oil
- - 1 tablespoon capers
- - 2 tablespoons fresh lemon juice
- - 2 cloves garlic, minced
- - Salt and pepper, to taste

Cooking method:
1. Preheat the oven to 400°F.
2. Place the cod filets in a baking dish.
3. In a small bowl, whisk together the olive oil, capers, lemon juice, garlic, salt, and pepper.
4. Pour the mixture over the cod filets and turn to coat.
5. Bake for 20 minutes, or until the cod is cooked through.

Turkey Burgers
Prep Time: 10 minutes | Cook Time: 10 minutes | Total Time: 20 minutes

INGREDIENTS:
- - 1 lb ground turkey
- - 1/2 cup breadcrumbs
- - 1/4 cup chopped onion
- - 1 teaspoon garlic powder
- - 1/2 teaspoon dried oregano

- - Salt and pepper, to taste
- - 4 whole wheat buns

Cooking method:
1. In a bowl, mix the ground turkey, breadcrumbs, onion, garlic powder, oregano, salt, and pepper until combined.
2. Form the mixture into 4 patties.
3. Heat a large skillet over medium-high heat.
4. Add the turkey patties to the skillet and cook on each side for 5 minutes, or until cooked through and no longer pink.
5. Serve the turkey patties on whole wheat buns.

Stuffed Sweet Potatoes
Prep Time: 10 minutes | Cook Time: 40 minutes | Total Time: 50 minutes

INGREDIENTS:

- - 4 sweet potatoes
- - 2 tablespoons olive oil
- - 1 can black beans, drained and rinsed
- - 1/4 cup diced red onion
- - 1/4 cup corn
- - 1/4 cup diced red bell pepper
- - 1/4 cup diced green bell pepper
- - 2 tablespoons chopped cilantro
- - Salt and pepper, to taste

Cooking method:
1. Preheat the oven to 400°F.
2. Prick the sweet potatoes several times with a fork.
3. Place the sweet potatoes on a baking sheet and drizzle with olive oil.
4. Bake for 40 minutes, or until the sweet potatoes are tender.
5. In a bowl, mix together the black beans, onion, corn, red bell pepper, green bell pepper, cilantro, salt, and pepper.

6. When the sweet potatoes are done, split them open and fill with the black bean mixture.
7. Serve.

Turkey Taco Bowls
Prep Time: 10 minutes | Cook Time: 20 minutes | Total Time: 30 minutes

INGREDIENTS:
- - 1 tablespoon olive oil
- - 1 lb ground turkey
- - 1 packet taco seasoning
- - 2 cups cooked brown rice
- - 1 can black beans, drained and rinsed
- - 1/2 cup salsa
- - 1/2 cup shredded cheddar cheese
- - 1/4 cup diced red onion
- - 1/4 cup diced tomatoes
- - 1/4 cup chopped fresh cilantro

- - Salt and pepper, to taste

Cooking method:
1. Heat the olive oil in a large skillet over medium-high heat.
2. Add the ground turkey and taco seasoning and cook for 8 minutes, or until the turkey is cooked through.
3. Place the cooked brown rice in a bowl and top with the cooked turkey, black beans, salsa, cheese, red onion, tomatoes, cilantro, salt, and pepper.
4. Serve.

Roasted Chicken And Vegetables
Prep Time: 10 minutes | Cook Time: 45 minutes | Total Time: 55 minutes

INGREDIENTS:
- - 4 boneless, skinless chicken breasts
- - 2 tablespoons olive oil

- - 1 red bell pepper, diced
- - 1 yellow bell pepper, diced
- - 1 zucchini, diced
- - 1 yellow squash, diced
- - 2 cloves garlic, minced
- - 1 teaspoon dried oregano
- - Salt and pepper, to taste

Cooking method:
1. Preheat the oven to 400°F.
2. Place the diced vegetables in a baking dish and drizzle with olive oil, garlic, oregano, salt, and pepper.
3. Place the chicken breasts on top of the vegetables and drizzle with olive oil, salt, and pepper.
4. Roast for 45 minutes.
5. Serve the chicken and roasted vegetables together.

Veggie Stir Fry

Prep Time: 10 minutes | Cook Time: 10 minutes | Total Time: 20 minutes

INGREDIENTS:
- - 2 tablespoons olive oil
- - 1 onion, diced
- - 2 carrots, sliced
- - 1 red bell pepper, diced
- - 1 yellow bell pepper, diced
- - 1 zucchini, diced
- - 1 yellow squash, diced
- - 2 cloves garlic, minced
- - 1 teaspoon freshly grated ginger
- - 2 tablespoons soy sauce
- - Salt and pepper, to taste

Cooking method:
1. Heat the olive oil in a large skillet over medium-high heat.
2. Add the onion, carrots, bell peppers, zucchini, yellow squash, garlic, and

ginger to the skillet and cook for 5 minutes.

3. Add the soy sauce, salt, and pepper and cook for an additional 3 minutes.

4. Serve.

Baked Salmon With Avocado Salsa

Prep Time: 10 minutes | Cook Time: 20 minutes | Total Time: 30 minutes

INGREDIENTS:
- - 4 4-ounce salmon filets
- - 2 tablespoons olive oil
- - Salt and pepper, to taste
- - 1 avocado, diced
- - 1/4 cup diced red onion
- - 1/4 cup diced tomatoes
- - 1/4 cup chopped fresh cilantro
- - 2 tablespoons freshly squeezed lime juice

Cooking method

1. Preheat the oven to 400°F.
2. Place the salmon filets on a baking sheet and drizzle with olive oil, salt, and pepper.
3. Bake for 20 minutes, or until the salmon is cooked through.
4. In a bowl, mix together the avocado, onion, tomatoes, cilantro, lime juice, salt, and pepper.
5. Serve the salmon with the avocado salsa.

Grilled Salmon with Garlic and Parsley
INGREDIENTS:

- 4 salmon filets, skin on
- 4 cloves garlic, minced
- 1/4 cup fresh parsley, chopped
- 2 tbsp olive oil
- Salt and pepper

Cooking method:
Preheat the grill to medium-high heat.
In a small bowl, mix together garlic,
parsley, olive oil, salt, and pepper.
Rub the garlic and parsley mixture onto
the salmon filets.
Grill salmon for 5-7 minutes per side or
until cooked to desired doneness.
Serve immediately.

Nutritional value per serving (based on 4
servings):
Calories: 319
Protein: 34g
Fat: 18g
Carbohydrates: 2g
Fiber: 1g
Sugar: 0g
Sodium: 102mg

Prep time: 10 minutes
Cook time: 10-14 minutes

Baked Chicken with Herbs and Lemon

INGREDIENTS:

- 4 boneless, skinless chicken breasts
- 2 tbsp olive oil
- 2 tbsp fresh lemon juice
- 2 cloves garlic, minced
- 1 tsp dried oregano
- 1 tsp dried thyme
- Salt and pepper

Cooking method:

Preheat the oven to 375°F.

In a small bowl, mix together olive oil, lemon juice, garlic, oregano, thyme, salt, and pepper.

Place chicken breasts in a baking dish and pour the herb and lemon mixture over the top.

Bake for 25-30 minutes or until chicken is cooked through.

Nutritional value per serving (based on 4 servings):

Calories: 265

Protein: 36g

Fat: 11g

Carbohydrates: 2g

Fiber: 0g

Sugar: 0g

Sodium: 160mg

Prep time: 10 minutes

Cook time: 25-30 minutes

Roasted Root Vegetables with Dill
INGREDIENTS:

- 2 medium sweet potatoes, peeled and cubed
- 2 medium beets, peeled and cubed
- 2 medium carrots, peeled and sliced

- 2 tbsp olive oil
- 2 tbsp fresh dill, chopped
- Salt and pepper

Cooking method:
Preheat the oven to 400°F.
In a large bowl, toss sweet potatoes, beets, and carrots with olive oil, dill, salt, and pepper.
Spread vegetables in a single layer on a baking sheet.
Roast for 25-30 minutes or until vegetables are tender and lightly browned.

Nutritional value per serving Calories: 142
Protein: 2g
Fat: 7g
Carbohydrates: 19g
Fiber: 4g
Sugar: 8g
Sodium: 132 mg

Prep time: 10 minutes
Cook time: 25-30 minutes

Grilled Fish Tacos with Cilantro Lime Slaw
INGREDIENTS:

- 1 pound white fish filets (such as tilapia or cod)
- 1 teaspoon chili powder
- 1/2 teaspoon cumin
- Salt and pepper to taste
- 8 small corn tortillas
- 2 cups shredded cabbage
- 1/4 cup chopped cilantro
- 1/4 cup mayonnaise
- 2 tablespoons lime juice
- 1 tablespoon honey

Cooking Method:
Preheat the grill to medium-high heat.
Season fish with chili powder, cumin,
salt, and pepper.

Grill fish for 4-5 minutes per side, or
until cooked through.

Warm tortillas on the grill for 30 seconds
per side.

In a medium bowl, mix together cabbage,
cilantro, mayonnaise, lime juice, and
honey.

Assemble tacos by placing fish on tortilla,
topped with slaw.

Nutritional Value:Calories: 295
Fat: 8g
Protein: 27g
Carbohydrates: 29g
Fiber: 5g

Sugar: 5g
Sodium: 354mg
Prep Time: 20 minutes

Zucchini Noodle Bowl with Pesto
INGREDIENTS:

-
- 4 medium zucchinis, spiralized into noodles
- 1/2 cup basil leaves
- 1/4 cup pine nuts
- 2 cloves garlic, minced
- 1/4 cup grated Parmesan cheese
- 1/4 cup olive oil
- Salt and pepper to taste
- 1/2 cup cherry tomatoes, halved
- 1/4 cup sliced black olives
- 1/4 cup crumbled feta cheese

Cooking Method:

In a food processor, combine basil, pine nuts, garlic, Parmesan cheese, olive oil, salt, and pepper. Process until smooth.
In a large bowl, toss zucchini noodles with pesto.
Top with cherry tomatoes, black olives, and feta cheese.

Nutritional Value:Calories: 330, Fat: 28g, Protein: 9g, Carbohydrates: 15g
Fiber: 5g
Sugar: 8g
Sodium: 375mg

Prep Time: 25 minutes

Baked Eggplant Parmesan
INGREDIENTS:

- 2 medium eggplants, sliced into 1/2-inch rounds
- Salt and pepper to taste

- 2 eggs, beaten
- 1 cup Italian seasoned breadcrumbs
- 1/2 cup grated Parmesan cheese
- 2 cups marinara sauce
- 1 cup shredded mozzarella cheese
- 1/4 cup chopped fresh basil

Cooking Method:
Preheat the oven to 375°F.
Season eggplant slices with salt and pepper.
Dip eggplant slices in beaten eggs, then coat in breadcrumbs mixed with Parmesan cheese.

Place eggplant slices on a baking sheet and bake for 20-25 minutes, or until golden brown.
In a 9x13 inch baking dish, spread a thin layer of marinara sauce.

Layer baked eggplant slices on top of the sauce.

Spoon remaining marinara sauce over the eggplant, and sprinkle with mozzarella cheese.
Bake for 25-30 minutes, or until the cheese is melted and bubbly.
Garnish with chopped fresh basil before serving.

Nutritional Value:
Calories: 385
Fat: 15g
Protein: 21

Lentil and Vegetable Stew
INGREDIENTS:
- 2 tablespoons olive oil
- 1 onion, chopped
- 2 cloves garlic, minced
- 2 carrots, chopped
- 2 celery stalks, chopped
- 1 red bell pepper, chopped
- 1 teaspoon ground cumin

- 1 teaspoon paprika
- 1/2 teaspoon ground coriander
- 1/4 teaspoon cayenne pepper
- 1 cup dried green lentils, rinsed and drained
- 4 cups vegetable broth
- 1 can (14.5 oz) diced tomatoes, undrained
- Salt and pepper to taste
- 1/4 cup chopped fresh parsley

Cooking Method:
In a large pot, heat olive oil over medium heat.
Add onion and garlic, and cook until onion is translucent, about 5 minutes.

Add carrots, celery, and red bell pepper, and cook for 5-7 minutes, until vegetables begin to soften.
Add cumin, paprika, coriander, and cayenne pepper, and cook for 1 minute, until fragrant.

Add lentils, vegetable broth, and tomatoes to the pot. Bring to a boil, then reduce heat to low and simmer for 30-35 minutes, until lentils are tender.
Season with salt and pepper to taste.
Ladle into bowls and garnish with chopped parsley.

Nutritional Value:,Calories: 225, Fat: 7g, Protein: 11g, Carbohydrates: 32g, Fiber: 13g
Sugar: 8g
Sodium: 754mg

Prep Time: 15 minutes
Cook Time: 45 minutes

Cauliflower Rice Stir Fry with Edamame

INGREDIENTS:
- 1 medium-sized cauliflower

- 1 cup shelled edamame
- 1 red bell pepper, diced
- 1 small onion, diced
- 2 cloves garlic, minced
- 2 tbsp olive oil
- 2 tbsp soy sauce
- 1 tbsp sesame oil
- Salt and pepper, to taste
- Chopped scallions, for garnish

Cooking method:
Cut the cauliflower into small florets and pulse in a food processor until it resembles rice.
In a large skillet, heat the olive oil over medium-high heat. Add the onion and red bell pepper and sauté until tender.
Add the minced garlic and cook for another minute.
Add the cauliflower rice and edamame and stir to combine.

Add soy sauce, sesame oil, salt, and pepper. Cook for 5-7 minutes or until the cauliflower is tender and slightly browned.
Garnish with chopped scallions and serve hot.

Nutritional Value (per serving):
Calories: 170 kcal | Carbohydrates: 13g | Protein: 8g | Fat: 11g | Saturated Fat: 1g | Sodium: 450mg | Fiber: 6g | Sugar: 4g

Prep Time: 15 minutes | Cook Time: 15 minutes

Slow Cooker Butternut Squash Soup
INGREDIENTS:
- 1 medium-sized butternut squash, peeled and diced
- 1 small onion, diced
- 2 cloves garlic, minced

- 2 cups chicken or vegetable broth
- 1 tsp ground cinnamon
- 1/2 tsp ground ginger
- 1/4 tsp ground nutmeg
- 1/4 tsp cayenne pepper (optional)
- Salt and pepper, to taste
- 1/4 cup heavy cream (optional)

Cooking method:
In a slow cooker, combine the diced butternut squash, onion, garlic, chicken or vegetable broth, cinnamon, ginger, nutmeg, cayenne pepper (if using), salt, and pepper.
Cook on high for 3-4 hours or low for 6-8 hours, or until the butternut squash is tender.

Using an immersion blender or a regular blender, blend the soup until smooth.
Stir in the heavy cream (if using) and adjust seasoning as needed.
Serve hot.

Nutritional Value (per serving):
Calories: 110 kcal | Carbohydrates: 19g |
Protein: 2g | Fat: 4g | Saturated Fat: 2g |
Sodium: 440mg | Fiber: 3g | Sugar: 5g

Prep Time: 15 minutes | Cook Time: 3-8
hours (depending on slow cooker setting)

Black Bean and Rice Burrito Bowl
INGREDIENTS:
- 1 cup cooked brown rice
- 1 can black beans, drained and rinsed
- 1 red bell pepper, diced
- 1 small onion, diced
- 1/2 cup frozen corn, thawed
- 1 avocado, diced
- 1/4 cup chopped fresh cilantro
- 2 tbsp olive oil
- 1 lime, juiced
- 1 tsp ground cumin

- Salt and pepper, to taste

Cooking method:
In a large bowl, combine the cooked brown rice, black beans, red bell pepper, onion, corn, avocado, and cilantro.

In a small bowl, whisk together the olive oil, lime juice, ground cumin, salt, and pepper.
Pour the dressing over the rice and bean mixture and toss to combine.
Serve hot or cold.

Nutritional Value (per serving):
Calories: 350 kcal | Carbohydrates: 45g | Protein: 10g | Fat: 16g | Saturated Fat: 2g | Sodium: 220mg | Fiber: 12g | Sugar: 3g

Prep Time: 10 minutes | Cook Time: 25 minutes (for brown rice)

Grilled Portobello Mushroom Burger

INGREDIENTS:

- 4 large portobello mushroom caps
- 1 red onion, sliced into thick rounds
- 4 whole wheat hamburger buns
- 4 slices provolone cheese
- 2 tbsp balsamic vinegar
- 2 tbsp olive oil
- 1 tsp dried thyme
- Salt and pepper, to taste
- Arugula or other greens, for serving

Cooking method:

Preheat a grill or grill pan over medium-high heat.

In a small bowl, whisk together the balsamic vinegar, olive oil, dried thyme, salt, and pepper.

Brush the portobello mushroom caps and red onion rounds with the balsamic mixture.

Grill the mushrooms and onions for 4-5 minutes per side or until tender.
During the last minute of grilling, top each mushroom cap with a slice of provolone cheese.
Toast the hamburger buns on the grill.

Assemble the burgers by placing a grilled mushroom cap on the bottom half of each bun, followed by a grilled red onion round and a handful of arugula or other greens. Top with the other half of the bun.
Serve hot.
Nutritional Value (per serving):
Calories: 300 kcal | Carbohydrates: 28g | Protein: 14g | Fat: 16g | Saturated Fat: 5g | Sodium

BLOOD PRESSURE DOWN DESSERT RECIPES

1. Banana Coconut Chia Pudding
INGREDIENTS
- - 2 cups unsweetened almond milk
- - 2 tablespoons chia seeds
- - 4 tablespoons maple syrup
- - 2 teaspoons pure vanilla extract
- - 2 ripe bananas
- - 2 tablespoons unsweetened coconut flakes

Cooking method:
1. In a medium bowl, whisk together almond milk, chia seeds, maple syrup, and vanilla extract.

2. Let sit for 10 minutes, stirring occasionally to keep clumps from forming.

3. In a separate bowl, mash the bananas until smooth.

4. Add the mashed bananas to the chia mixture and stir until combined.

5. Divide the pudding among 4 glass jars or containers and top each with 1/2 tablespoon of coconut flakes.

6. Refrigerate for at least 1 hour before serving.

2. Apple Peach Crisp
INGREDIENTS
- 2 cups diced apples
- - 2 cups diced peaches
- - 2 tablespoons honey
- - 2 tablespoons lemon juice
- - 2 tablespoons cornstarch
- - 2 tablespoons coconut oil

- - 1/2 teaspoon ground cinnamon
- - 1/4 teaspoon ground nutmeg
- - 1/4 cup rolled oats
- - 1/4 cup almond flour
- - 1/4 teaspoon sea salt

Cooking method:
1. Preheat the oven to 350°F.

2. In a medium bowl, combine apples, peaches, honey, lemon juice, and cornstarch. Stir until the fruit is thoroughly coated.

3. Pour the mixture into a 9-inch baking dish and spread evenly.

4. In a small bowl, combine coconut oil, cinnamon, nutmeg, oats, almond flour, and sea salt. Stir until everything is combined.

5. Sprinkle the topping over the fruit mixture and spread evenly.

6. Bake for 25-30 minutes or until the topping is golden brown and the fruit is bubbly.

7. Let cool for 10 minutes before serving. Enjoy!

3. Baked Apples
INGREDIENTS
- - 4 apples, cored and halved
- - 2 tablespoons maple syrup
- - 2 tablespoons walnuts, chopped
- - 2 tablespoons coconut flakes
- - 1/2 teaspoon ground cinnamon
- - 1/4 teaspoon ground nutmeg
- - Pinch of sea salt

Cooking method:
1. Preheat the oven to 350°F.

2. Place the apples cut-side up in an oven-safe baking dish.

3. Drizzle maple syrup over the apples and sprinkle with walnuts, coconut flakes, cinnamon, nutmeg, and sea salt.

4. Bake for 25-30 minutes or until the apples are tender.

5. Let cool for 10 minutes before serving. Enjoy!

4. Baked Pears With Cinnamon
INGREDIENTS
- - 4 pears, cored and halved
- - 2 tablespoons maple syrup
- - 2 tablespoons walnuts, chopped
- - 2 tablespoons coconut flakes
- - 1/2 teaspoon ground cinnamon
- - 1/4 teaspoon ground nutmeg

- - Pinch of sea salt

Cooking method:
1. Preheat the oven to 350°F.

2. Place the pears cut-side up in an oven-safe baking dish.

3. Drizzle maple syrup over the pears and sprinkle with walnuts, coconut flakes, cinnamon, nutmeg, and sea salt.

4. Bake for 25-30 minutes or until the pears are tender.

5. Let cool for 10 minutes before serving. Enjoy!

5. Banana Split Parfaits
INGREDIENTS
- - 2 bananas, sliced
- - 2 tablespoons chocolate syrup

- - 2 tablespoons walnuts, chopped
- - 2 tablespoons coconut flakes
- - 1/2 teaspoon ground cinnamon
- - 2 cups plain Greek yogurt

Cooking method:
1. Layer the banana slices, chocolate syrup, walnuts, coconut flakes, and cinnamon in the bottom of 4 glasses.

2. Top with the Greek yogurt and repeat the layering process.

3. Refrigerate until ready to serve. Enjoy!

6. Fruit Salad With Yogurt
INGREDIENTS
- - 2 cups diced apples
- - 2 cups diced peaches
- - 2 cups diced strawberries
- - 2 tablespoons honey

- - 2 tablespoons lemon juice
- - 2 cups plain Greek yogurt

Cooking method:
1. In a large bowl, combine apples, peaches, and strawberries.

2. Drizzle with honey and lemon juice and stir until the fruit is thoroughly coated.

3. Divide the mixture among 4 bowls and top each with 1/2 cup of Greek yogurt.

4. Enjoy!

7. Oatmeal Cookies
INGREDIENTS
- - 2 cups rolled oats
- - 1/2 cup almond flour
- - 2 tablespoons coconut oil
- - 1/4 cup honey

- - 1/4 teaspoon ground cinnamon
- - 1/4 teaspoon sea salt

Cooking method:
1. Preheat the oven to 350°F.

2. In a medium bowl, combine oats, almond flour, coconut oil, honey, cinnamon, and sea salt. Stir until everything is combined.

3. Drop tablespoon-sized balls of dough onto a parchment-lined baking sheet.

4. Bake for 10-12 minutes or until the cookies are golden brown.

5. Let cool for 10 minutes before serving. Enjoy!

8. Chocolate Coconut Mousse
INGREDIENTS

- - 2 ripe avocados
- - 1/4 cup cocoa powder
- - 2 tablespoons maple syrup
- - 2 tablespoons coconut flakes
- - 1 teaspoon pure vanilla extract

Cooking method:
1. In a food processor or blender, combine avocados, cocoa powder, maple syrup, coconut flakes, and vanilla extract. Blend until smooth.

2. Divide the mousse among 4 small bowls.

3. Refrigerate for 1 hour before serving. Enjoy!

9. Frozen Yogurt Bark
INGREDIENTS
- - 2 cups plain Greek yogurt
- - 2 tablespoons honey

- - 2 tablespoons coconut flakes
- - 2 tablespoons walnuts, chopped
- - 1/2 teaspoon ground cinnamon

Cooking method:
1. Line a baking sheet with parchment paper.

2. In a medium bowl, combine yogurt, honey, coconut flakes, walnuts, and cinnamon. Stir until everything is combined.

3. Spread the mixture onto the parchment-lined baking sheet, forming a single layer.

4. Place in the freezer for 1 hour or until firm.

5. Break into pieces and enjoy!

10. Coconut Macaroons

INGREDIENTS

- - 2 cups unsweetened shredded coconut
- - 2 tablespoons honey
- - 2 tablespoons coconut oil
- - 1 teaspoon pure vanilla extract
- - Pinch of sea salt

Cooking method:

1. Preheat the oven to 350°F.

2. In a medium bowl, combine coconut, honey, coconut oil, vanilla extract, and sea salt. Stir until everything is combined.

3. Drop tablespoon-sized balls of dough onto a parchment-lined baking sheet.

4. Bake for 10-12 minutes or until the cookies are golden brown.

5. Let cool for 10 minutes before serving. Enjoy!

CHAPTER 3: HEALTHY SNACK OPTIONS

1. Air-popped Popcorn

INGREDIENTS:

- - 2 tablespoons popcorn kernels
- - 1 teaspoon olive oil
- - Herbs and spices to taste

Cooking method:

1. In a large pot, heat the olive oil over medium heat.

2. Add the popcorn kernels and cover the pot with a lid.

3. Shake the pot gently so that the popcorn kernels are evenly distributed in the oil.

4. Once the popcorn starts to pop, reduce the heat to low and continue to shake the pot.

5. When the popping slows down, remove the pot from heat and pour the popcorn into a bowl.
6. Add herbs and spices to taste and serve.

2. Baked Apple Slices with Cinnamon
INGREDIENTS:
- - 2 apples, peeled and sliced
- - 2 tablespoons maple syrup
- - 1 teaspoon ground cinnamon
- - 1/4 teaspoon ground nutmeg

Cooking method:
1. Preheat the oven to 350°F.
2. Arrange the apple slices in a single layer on a baking sheet.
3. In a small bowl, mix together the maple syrup, cinnamon, and nutmeg.

4. Drizzle the mixture over the apple slices and toss to coat.
5. Bake for 15 minutes, or until the apples are tender.
6. Serve warm.

3. Celery Sticks with Hummus
INGREDIENTS:
- - 2 stalks celery, sliced into sticks
- - 1/2 cup hummus
- - 1/4 teaspoon garlic powder

Cooking method:
1. Arrange the celery sticks on a plate.
2. In a small bowl, mix together the hummus and garlic powder.
3. Spread the hummus onto the celery sticks.
4. Serve.

4. Hard-Boiled Eggs
INGREDIENTS:
- - 6 eggs
- - 1 teaspoon olive oil

Cooking method:
1. Heat the olive oil in a medium pot over medium heat.
2. Carefully add the eggs to the pot and cover with a lid.
3. Reduce the heat to low and let the eggs cook for 8-10 minutes.
4. Remove the eggs from the pot and transfer to a bowl of cold water.
5. Peel the eggs and serve.

5. Roasted Chickpeas
INGREDIENTS:
- - 1 can chickpeas, rinsed and drained
- - 1 tablespoon olive oil
- - 1 teaspoon garlic powder

- - 1/4 teaspoon smoked paprika

Cooking method:
1. Preheat the oven to 400°F.
2. Arrange the chickpeas on a baking sheet.
3. Drizzle with olive oil and sprinkle with garlic powder and smoked paprika.
4. Roast for 20-25 minutes, or until the chickpeas are crispy.
5. Serve.

6. Greek Yogurt with Berries
INGREDIENTS:
- - 1 cup Greek yogurt
- - 1/2 cup fresh berries
- - 1 tablespoon honey

Cooking method:
1. In a bowl, mix together the Greek yogurt, berries, and honey.
2. Serve.

7. Edamame
INGREDIENTS:
- - 2 cups edamame, shelled
- - 1/4 teaspoon garlic powder
- - 1/4 teaspoon sea salt

Cooking method:
1. Bring a pot of salted water to a boil.
2. Add the edamame and cook for 5 minutes.
3. Drain the edamame and transfer to a bowl.
4. Sprinkle it with garlic powder and sea salt.
5. Serve.

8. Carrot Sticks with Guacamole
INGREDIENTS:
- - 4 carrots, sliced into sticks
- - 1/2 cup guacamole

- - 1/4 teaspoon ground cumin

Cooking method:
1. Arrange the carrot sticks on a plate.
2. In a small bowl, mix together the guacamole and cumin.
3. Spread the guacamole onto the carrot sticks.
4. Serve.

9. Whole-Grain Crackers with Peanut Butter

INGREDIENTS:
- - 8 whole-grain crackers
- - 2 tablespoons natural peanut butter
- - 1 teaspoon honey

Cooking method:
1. Spread the peanut butter onto the crackers.
2. Drizzle with honey.

3. Serve.

10. Fruit and Nut Mix
INGREDIENTS:
- - 1/2 cup dried fruit, chopped
- - 1/4 cup nuts
- - 1/2 teaspoon ground cinnamon

Instructions:
1. In a bowl, mix together the dried fruit, nuts, and cinnamon.
2. Serve.

11. Trail Mix:
INGREDIENTS:
- ½ cup roasted, unsalted almonds,
- ½ cup roasted, unsalted walnuts,
- ¼ cup dried cranberries,
- ¼ cup dark chocolate chips,
- ¼ cup sunflower seeds

Cooking Method:
Mix all ingredients together
Prep Time: 5 minutes

Nutritional Value: Calories: 545, Protein: 17g, Fat: 39g, Carbs: 34g, Fiber: 8g

12. Oatmeal with Nuts and Honey:
INGREDIENTS:
- 1 cup rolled oats,
- 2 cups water,
- 1 tablespoon honey,
- 2 tablespoons chopped almonds

Cooking Method:
Bring the water to a boil in a medium saucepan. Stir in the oats and reduce the heat to medium-low.

Simmer until the oats are tender, about 5 minutes. Add the honey and almonds, stirring to combine.
Cooking Time: 10 minutes

Nutritional Value: Calories: 286, Protein: 9g, Fat: 8g, Carbs: 45g, Fiber: 6g

13. Cottage Cheese with Fruits:
INGREDIENTS:
- ½ cup low-fat cottage cheese,
- ½ cup berries of choice,
- 2 tablespoons chopped walnuts

Cooking Method:
Mix all ingredients together.
Prep Time: 5 minutes

Nutritional Value: Calories: 124, Protein: 9g, Fat: 6g, Carbs: 10g, Fiber: 2g

14. Whole-Grain Toast with Avocado:

INGREDIENTS:

- 2 slices whole-grain bread,
- ½ avocado, sliced, pinch of salt

Cooking Method:
Toast the bread.
Spread the avocado on the toast and sprinkle with a pinch of salt.
Cooking Time: 5 minutes

Nutritional Value: Calories: 277, Protein: 7g, Fat: 14g, Carbs: 33g, Fiber: 7g

15. Rice Cakes with Nut Butter:

INGREDIENTS:

- 2 rice cakes,
- 2 tablespoons nut butter of choice

Cooking Method:
Spread the nut butter on the rice cakes.
Prep Time: 5 minutes

Nutritional Value: Calories: 220, Protein: 6g, Fat: 13g, Carbs: 21g, Fiber: 1g

16. Low-Fat Popcorn:
INGREDIENTS:
- 4 cups air-popped popcorn

Cooking Method:
Heat a large pot over medium heat.
Add the popcorn kernels and cover.
Shake the pot occasionally until the kernels have all popped.
Transfer the popcorn to a bowl and enjoy.
Prep Time: 5 minutes

Nutritional Value: Calories: 109, Protein: 3g, Fat: 2g, Carbs: 21g, Fiber: 4g

17. Low-Fat Cheese and Whole-Grain Crackers:

INGREDIENTS:

- 4 ounces low-fat cheese,
- 10 whole-grain crackers

Cooking Method:
Cut the cheese into cubes and serve with the crackers.
Prep Time: 5 minutes

Nutritional Value: Calories: 300, Protein: 16g, Fat: 13g, Carbs: 30g, Fiber: 5g

18. Low-Fat Yogurt with Granola:

INGREDIENTS:

- 1 cup low-fat yogurt,
- ¼ cup granola

Cooking Method:
Mix the yogurt and granola together.
Prep Time: 5 minutes

Nutritional Value: Calories: 173, Protein: 10g, Fat: 2g, Carbs: 29g, Fiber: 2g

19. Veggies and Low-Fat Dip:
INGREDIENTS:
- 1 cup of raw vegetables of choice,
- ¼ cup low-fat dip

Cooking Method:
Arrange the vegetables on a plate and serve with the dip.
Prep Time: 10 minutes

Nutritional Value: Calories: 95, Protein: 3g, Fat: 5g, Carbs: 9g, Fiber: 3g

20. Fresh Fruit Smoothie:

INGREDIENTS:

- 1 cup frozen fruit of choice,
- 1 banana,
- ½ cup almond milk,
- 2 tablespoons honey

Cooking Method:
Place the fruit, banana, almond milk, and honey in a blender. Blend until smooth.
Prep Time: 5 minutes

Nutritional Value: Calories: 186, Protein: 2g, Fat: 2g, Carbs: 43g, Fiber: 4g

BEVERAGES TO PROMOTE HEALTHY BLOOD PRESSURE

1. Beet, Carrot, and Orange Juice
INGREDIENTS:
- 2 medium-sized beets
- 2 small carrots
- 2 oranges

Cooking Method:
1. Wash the beets and carrots and peel the oranges.
2. Cut the beets and carrots into small pieces and place them into a juicer.
3. Juice the oranges and add them to the juicer.
4. Turn the juicer on and blend until it is a smooth, liquid juice.

Prep Time: 10 minutes

Nutritional Value: Calcium, vitamin C, vitamin A, vitamin B6, iron, and magnesium

2. Pomegranate Green Tea
INGREDIENTS:

- 2 tablespoons of green tea
- ½ cup of boiling water
- 1 tablespoon of pomegranate juice
- ½ teaspoon of honey

Cooking Method:
1. Boil the water in a small pot.
2. Add the green tea to the boiling water and let it steep for 5 minutes.
3. Strain the tea into a cup and add the pomegranate juice and honey.
4. Stir the tea until the honey is dissolved and enjoy.

Prep Time: 10 minutes

Nutritional Value: Antioxidants, vitamin C, and vitamin K

3. Watermelon and Basil Infused Water

INGREDIENTS:
- 2 cups of watermelon chunks
- 2 tablespoons of fresh basil leaves
- 2 cups of cold water

Cooking Method:
1. Place the watermelon chunks and basil leaves in a pitcher.
2. Pour the cold water into the pitcher and let it sit for 30 minutes.
3. Strain the watermelon chunks and basil leaves and enjoy.

Prep Time: 10 minutes
Nutritional Value: Vitamin A, vitamin C, and magnesium

4. Blueberry and Coconut Milk Smoothie

INGREDIENTS:

- ½ cup of frozen blueberries
- ¾ cup of coconut milk
- 1 tablespoon of chia seeds
- 1 teaspoon of honey

Cooking Method:

1. Place the frozen blueberries, coconut milk, chia seeds, and honey in a blender.
2. Blend until it is a smooth, creamy consistency.
3. Pour the smoothie into a glass and enjoy.

Prep Time: 5 minutes
Nutritional Value: Protein, fiber, vitamin C, vitamin K, and potassium

5. Strawberry and Banana Smoothie

INGREDIENTS:

- 1 banana
- ½ cup of frozen strawberries
- ½ cup of almond milk
- 1 teaspoon of honey

Cooking Method:

1. Peel the banana and place it in a blender.
2. Add the frozen strawberries, almond milk, and honey.
3. Blend until it is a smooth, creamy consistency.
4. Pour the smoothie into a glass and enjoy.

Prep Time: 5 minutes
Nutritional Value: Vitamin C, vitamin B6, potassium, and magnesium

6. Apple Cider Vinegar and Honey Drink

INGREDIENTS:

- 2 tablespoons of apple cider vinegar
- 1 teaspoon of honey
- 1 cup of warm water

Cooking Method:

1. Place the apple cider vinegar and honey in a cup.
2. Pour the warm water into the cup and stir until the honey is dissolved.
3. Enjoy the drink.

Prep Time: 5 minutes
Nutritional Value: Acetic acid, potassium, and amino acids

7. Chia Seed and Avocado Smoothie

INGREDIENTS:

- ½ avocado
- ¼ cup of chia seeds
- 1 cup of almond milk
- 1 teaspoon of honey

Cooking Method:
1. Cut the avocado in half and scoop out the flesh.
2. Place the avocado and chia seeds in a blender.
3. Add the almond milk and honey.
4. Blend until it is a smooth, creamy consistency.
5. Pour the smoothie into a glass and enjoy.

Prep Time: 5 minutes
Nutritional Value: Protein, fiber, vitamin C, vitamin E, and omega-3 fatty acids

8. Green Tea with Lemon and Ginger

INGREDIENTS:
- 1 teaspoon of green tea leaves
- ½ cup of boiling water
- 1 teaspoon of freshly grated ginger
- 1 teaspoon of freshly squeezed lemon juice

Cooking Method:
1. Boil the water in a small pot.
2. Add the green tea leaves to the boiling water and let it steep for 5 minutes.
3. Strain the tea into a cup and add the ginger and lemon juice.
4. Stir the tea until the ginger and lemon juice are dissolved and enjoy.

Prep Time: 10 minutes
Nutritional Value: Antioxidants, vitamin C, and vitamin B6

9. Tart Cherry Juice
INGREDIENTS:

- 2 cups of tart cherries
- 2 tablespoons of honey
- 1 cup of water

Cooking Method:
1. Place the tart cherries in a blender.
2. Add the honey and water.
3. Blend until it is a smooth, liquid juice.
4. Strain the juice into a glass and enjoy.

Prep Time: 10 minutes
Nutritional Value: Vitamin A, vitamin C, iron, and magnesium

10. Cucumber, Kale, and Celery Juice
INGREDIENTS:
- ½ cucumber
- 2 kale leaves
- 2 stalks of celery
- ½ cup of water

Cooking Method:
1. Wash the cucumber, kale, and celery.
2. Cut the cucumber and celery into small pieces and place them into a juicer.
3. Juice the kale and add it to the juicer.
4. Pour the water into the juicer and blend until it is a smooth, liquid juice.

11. Unsweetened Coconut Water
INGREDIENTS:
- - 1 coconut
- - 2 cups of water
- - 1 lime
- - 1 tablespoon of honey (optional)

Cooking Method:
1. Start by cutting the coconut in half and removing the meat from the inside.
2. Place the coconut meat in a blender and add the water.
3. Blend the mixture until it is a smooth liquid.

4. Strain the mixture through a sieve to remove any chunks.

5. Add the juice of one lime and honey (if desired) to the mixture.

6. Refrigerate the coconut water until chilled.

Nutritional Value:
Calories: 35
Carbohydrates: 6g
Protein: 1g
Fat: 0g
Fiber: 0g
Prep Time: 10 minutes

12. Turmeric and Almond Milk
INGREDIENTS:
- - 1 cup of almond milk
- - 1 teaspoon of turmeric powder
- - 1 tablespoon of honey (optional)

Cooking Method:

1. In a small saucepan, heat the almond milk over low heat.
2. Once the almond milk is heated, add the turmeric powder and stir until combined.
3. Remove the saucepan from the heat and add the honey (if desired).
4. Strain the mixture through a sieve to remove any chunks.
5. Refrigerate the almond milk until chilled.

Nutritional Value:
Calories: 81
Carbohydrates: 7g
Protein: 2g
Fat: 5g
Fiber: 0g

Prep Time: 10 minutes

13. Pineapple and Coconut Water Smoothie

INGREDIENTS:

- - 2 cups of unsweetened coconut water
- - 1 cup of fresh pineapple, diced
- - 1 banana, peeled and sliced
- - 1 tablespoon of honey (optional)

Cooking Method:

1. Place the coconut water, pineapple, and banana in a blender and blend until smooth.
2. Add the honey (if desired) and blend for an additional 30 seconds.
3. Pour the smoothie into glasses and serve.

Nutritional Value:
Calories: 162
Carbohydrates: 37g
Protein: 2g
Fat: 1g

Fiber: 3g
Prep Time: 5 minutes

14. Beet, Carrot, and Apple Juice

INGREDIENTS:

- - 2 beets, peeled and diced
- - 2 carrots, peeled and diced
- - 1 apple, peeled and diced
- - 1 cup of water

Cooking Method:
1. Place the beets, carrots, and apple in a juicer and juice until smooth.
2. Add the water and stir to combine.
3. Strain the mixture through a sieve to remove any chunks.
4. Refrigerate the juice until chilled.

Nutritional Value:
Calories: 111
Carbohydrates: 27g
Protein: 3g

Fat: 0g
Fiber: 7g
Prep Time: 10 minutes

15. Hibiscus Tea with Lime

INGREDIENTS:

- - 2 cups of water
- - 2 tablespoons of dried hibiscus flowers
- - 2 tablespoons of honey (optional)
- - 1 lime, juiced

Cooking Method:
1. In a small saucepan, heat the water over low heat.
2. Once the water is heated, add the hibiscus flowers and stir until combined.
3. Remove the saucepan from the heat and add the honey (if desired).
4. Strain the mixture through a sieve to remove any chunks.

5. Add the juice of one lime to the mixture.

6. Refrigerate the tea until chilled.

Nutritional Value:
Calories: 25
Carbohydrates: 6g
Protein: 0g
Fat: 0g
Fiber: 0g
Prep Time: 10 minutes

CHAPTER 4: SALAD AND SIDES

Cucumber and Tomato Salad
INGREDIENTS:
- 2 cucumbers,
- 4 tomatoes,
- 2 tablespoons of olive oil,
- 2 tablespoons of vinegar,
- 1 teaspoon of sugar, salt, and pepper to taste.

Prep Time: 10 minutes

Cooking Method:
Chop the cucumbers and tomatoes into small pieces and combine in a bowl.
Mix the olive oil, vinegar, sugar, salt, and pepper together in a separate bowl and pour over the cucumber and tomato mixture.
Toss and serve.

Nutritional Value: Low in calories and high in vitamins A, C, and K.

Kale and Avocado Salad
INGREDIENTS:
- 2 cups of kale,
- 2 avocados,
- 1 tablespoon of olive oil,
- 1 tablespoon of lemon juice,
- 1 teaspoon of garlic powder, salt, and pepper to taste.

Prep Time: 10 minutes

Cooking Method:
Massage the kale with the olive oil, lemon juice, garlic powder, salt, and pepper until wilted.
Slice the avocados and combine with the kale. Serve.

Nutritional Value: Low in calories and high in vitamins A, C, K, and E.

Quinoa and Chickpea Salad

INGREDIENTS:

- 1 cup of cooked quinoa,
- 1 cup of cooked chickpeas,
- 1/4 cup of diced red onion,
- 1/4 cup of diced red bell pepper,
- 1/4 cup of diced cucumber,
- 1/4 cup of diced tomatoes,
- 2 tablespoons of olive oil,
- 1 tablespoon of lemon juice,
- 1 teaspoon of garlic powder, salt, and pepper to taste.

Prep Time: 10 minutes

Cooking Method:
Combine all the ingredients in a bowl and toss until mixed. Serve.

Nutritional Value: Low in calories and high in protein, fiber, vitamins, and minerals.

Roasted Beet Salad
INGREDIENTS:
- 2 beets,
- 2 tablespoons of olive oil,
- 1 tablespoon of balsamic vinegar,
- 1 teaspoon of sugar, salt, and pepper to taste.

Prep Time: 15 minutes

Cooking Method:
Preheat the oven to 400 degrees F. Wash and cut beets into cubes.
Place on a baking sheet, drizzle with olive oil, balsamic vinegar, sugar, salt, and pepper.
Roast for 20 minutes. Remove from the oven and let cool. Serve.

Nutritional Value: Low in calories and high in vitamins A, C, and fiber.

Spinach and Feta Salad

INGREDIENTS:

- 2 cups of spinach,
- 1/4 cup of feta cheese,
- 1/4 cup of diced tomatoes,
- 1/4 cup of diced cucumber,
- 2 tablespoons of olive oil,
- 1 tablespoon of lemon juice,
- 1 teaspoon of garlic powder, salt, and pepper to taste.

Prep Time: 10 minutes

Cooking Method:
Combine all the ingredients in a bowl and toss until mixed. Serve.

Nutritional Value: Low in calories and high in vitamins A and C.

Lentil and Sweet Potato Salad

INGREDIENTS:

- 1 cup of cooked lentils,
- 1 sweet potato,
- 2 tablespoons of olive oil,
- 1 tablespoon of lemon juice,
- 1 teaspoon of garlic powder, salt, and pepper to taste.

Prep Time: 15 minutes

Cooking Method:

Preheat the oven to 400 degrees F. Wash and cut the sweet potato into cubes. Place on a baking sheet, drizzle with olive oil, lemon juice, garlic powder, salt, and pepper.

Roast for 20 minutes. Remove from oven and let cool. Combine cooked lentils and sweet potatoes in a bowl and toss until mixed. Serve.

Nutritional Value: Low in calories and high in protein, fiber, vitamins, and minerals.

Greek Salad
INGREDIENTS:
- 2 cups of lettuce,
- 1/4 cup of diced red onion,
- 1/4 cup of diced cucumber,
- 1/4 cup of diced tomatoes,
- 1/4 cup of chopped olives,
- 1/4 cup of feta cheese,
- 2 tablespoons of olive oil,
- 1 tablespoon of lemon juice,
- 1 teaspoon of oregano, salt, and pepper to taste.

Prep Time: 10 minutes

Cooking Method:

Combine all the ingredients in a bowl and toss until mixed. Serve.

Nutritional Value: Low in calories and high in vitamins A, C, K, and fiber.

Broccoli and Carrot Salad
INGREDIENTS:
- 2 cups of broccoli,
- 2 carrots,
- 2 tablespoons of olive oil,
- 1 tablespoon of apple cider vinegar,
- 1 teaspoon of honey, salt, and pepper to taste.

Prep Time: 10 minutes

Cooking Method:
Chop the broccoli and carrots into small pieces and combine in a bowl.

Mix the olive oil, vinegar, honey, salt, and pepper together in a separate bowl and

pour over the broccoli and carrot mixture.
Toss and serve.

Nutritional Value: Low in calories and high in vitamins A, C, and K.

Roasted Vegetable Salad
INGREDIENTS:
- 2 cups of mixed vegetables (such as zucchini, bell peppers, broccoli, and carrots),
- 2 tablespoons of olive oil,
- 1 tablespoon of balsamic vinegar,
- 1 teaspoon of sugar, salt, and pepper to taste.

Prep Time: 15 minutes

Cooking Method:
Preheat the oven to 400 degrees F. Wash and cut vegetables into cubes.

Place on a baking sheet, drizzle with olive oil, balsamic vinegar, sugar, salt, and pepper.

Roast for 20 minutes. Remove from the oven and let cool. Serve.

Nutritional Value: Low in calories and high in vitamins A, C, and fiber.

Spinach and Apple Salad

INGREDIENTS:
- 2 cups of spinach,
- 1 apple,
- 2 tablespoons of olive oil,
- 1 tablespoon of lemon juice,
- 1 teaspoon of honey, salt, and pepper to taste.

Prep Time: 10 minutes

Cooking Method:

Chop the apple into small pieces and combine with the spinach in a bowl.

Mix the olive oil, lemon juice, honey, salt, and pepper together in a separate bowl and pour over the spinach and apple mixture.

Toss and serve.

Nutritional Value: Low in calories and high in vitamins A and C.

Fruit and Nut Salad

INGREDIENTS:

- ½ cup walnuts,
- 2 tablespoons honey,
- 1 teaspoon cinnamon,
- 2 tablespoons olive oil,
- 2 cups fresh fruit of your choice (strawberries, blueberries, banana, pineapple, etc.),
- 2 tablespoons raisins

Cooking Method:

Preheat the oven to 350°F. Spread walnuts on a baking sheet lined with parchment paper and bake for 8-10 minutes, stirring once halfway through.

Meanwhile, in a small bowl, whisk together honey, cinnamon, and olive oil until combined. Once walnuts are done baking and cooled, combine with honey mixture, fresh fruit, and raisins in a large bowl and mix until evenly coated.

Prep Time: 10 minutes

Nutritional Value (per serving): Calories: 145; Total Fat: 9g; Saturated Fat: 1g; Cholesterol: 0mg; Sodium: 0mg; Total Carbohydrates: 15g; Dietary Fiber: 2g; Protein: 3g

Cauliflower and Broccoli Slaw

INGREDIENTS:

- 1 medium head cauliflower,
- 1 medium head broccoli,
- 2 tablespoons olive oil,
- 2 tablespoons balsamic vinegar,
- 2 tablespoons honey,
- 2 tablespoons fresh lemon juice,
- 1 teaspoon garlic powder

Cooking Method:
Preheat the oven to 400°F. Cut cauliflower and broccoli into small florets, discarding stalks.

Place florets on a baking sheet lined with parchment paper, drizzle with olive oil, and season with salt and pepper. Bake for 20-25 minutes, stirring once halfway through.

Meanwhile, in a small bowl, whisk together balsamic vinegar, honey, lemon juice, and garlic powder. Once vegetables are done baking, transfer to a large bowl and drizzle with honey mixture. Mix until evenly coated.

Prep Time: 15 minutes

Nutritional Value (per serving): Calories: 100; Total Fat: 5g; Saturated Fat: 1g; Cholesterol: 0mg; Sodium: 0mg; Total Carbohydrates: 12g; Dietary Fiber: 4g; Protein: 4g

Roasted Sweet Potato and Zucchini
INGREDIENTS:
- 2 large sweet potatoes,
- 2 medium zucchini,
- 2 tablespoons olive oil,
- 1 teaspoon garlic powder,
- 1 teaspoon dried oregano

Cooking Method:

Preheat the oven to 400°F. Peel and cube sweet potatoes.

Slice zucchini into thin rounds.

Place both vegetables on a baking sheet lined with parchment paper, drizzle with olive oil, and season with garlic powder, oregano, salt, and pepper.

Bake for 20-25 minutes, stirring once halfway through.

Prep Time: 10 minutes

Nutritional Value (per serving): Calories: 140; Total Fat: 7g; Saturated Fat: 1g; Cholesterol: 0mg; Sodium: 0mg; Total Carbohydrates: 18g; Dietary Fiber: 4g; Protein: 3g

Baked Zucchini Fries

INGREDIENTS:

- 2 medium zucchinis,
- ½ cup breadcrumbs,

- 2 tablespoons grated Parmesan cheese,
- 2 tablespoons olive oil,
- 1 teaspoon garlic powder

Cooking Method:
Preheat the oven to 400°F. Slice zucchinis into thin strips. In a shallow bowl, combine breadcrumbs, Parmesan cheese, garlic powder, and salt.

Drizzle with olive oil and mix until combined. Dip zucchini strips into breadcrumb mixture, coating evenly. Place on a baking sheet lined with parchment paper and bake for 20-25 minutes, flipping once halfway through.
Prep Time: 10 minutes

Nutritional Value (per serving): Calories: 90; Total Fat: 5g; Saturated Fat: 1g; Cholesterol: 2mg; Sodium: 140mg; Total

Carbohydrates: 9g; Dietary Fiber: 2g;
Protein: 3g

Roasted Brussels Sprouts

INGREDIENTS:

- 1 pound Brussels sprouts,
- 2 tablespoons olive oil,
- 1 teaspoon garlic powder,
- 1 teaspoon dried oregano

Cooking Method:
Preheat the oven to 400°F.
Trim ends off Brussels sprouts and slice in half. Place on a baking sheet lined with parchment paper, drizzle with olive oil, and season with garlic powder, oregano, salt, and pepper.

Bake for 20-25 minutes, stirring halfway through.
Prep Time: 10 minutes

Nutritional Value (per serving): Calories: 70; Total Fat: 4g; Saturated Fat: 1g; Cholesterol: 0mg; Sodium: 0mg; Total Carbohydrates: 8g; Dietary Fiber: 3g; Protein: 3g

Baked Sweet Potato Wedges
INGREDIENTS:
- 2 large sweet potatoes,
- 2 tablespoons olive oil,
- 1 teaspoon garlic powder

Cooking Method:
Preheat the oven to 400°F.
Peel and cut sweet potatoes into wedges. Place on a baking sheet lined with parchment paper, drizzle with olive oil, and season with garlic powder, salt, and pepper.

Bake for 20-25 minutes, flipping once
halfway through.
Prep Time: 10 minutes

Nutritional Value (per serving): Calories:
120; Total Fat: 5g; Saturated Fat: 1g;
Cholesterol: 0mg; Sodium: 0mg; Total
Carbohydrates: 18g; Dietary Fiber: 3g;
Protein: 2g

Baked Eggplant with Herbs

INGREDIENTS:

- 1 large eggplant,
- 2 tablespoons olive oil,
- 1 teaspoon dried oregano,
- 1 teaspoon dried basil,
- 1 teaspoon garlic powder

Cooking Method:
Preheat the oven to 400°F. Slice eggplant
into thick rounds. Place on a baking sheet

lined with parchment paper, drizzle with olive oil, and season with oregano, basil, garlic powder, salt, and pepper.
Bake for 20-25 minutes, flipping once halfway through.
Prep Time: 10 minutes

Nutritional Value (per serving): Calories: 80; Total Fat: 5g; Saturated Fat: 1g; Cholesterol: 0mg; Sodium: 0mg; Total Carbohydrates: 8g; Dietary Fiber: 3g; Protein: 2g

Baked Kale Chips
INGREDIENTS:
- 2 bunches kale,
- 2 tablespoons olive oil,
- 1 teaspoon garlic powder

Cooking Method:

Preheat the oven to 350°F. Remove kale leaves from stems and tear into bite-sized pieces.
Place on a baking sheet lined with parchment paper, drizzle with olive oil, and season with garlic powder, salt, and pepper.

Bake for 8-10 minutes, stirring once halfway through.
Prep Time: 10 minutes

Nutritional Value (per serving): Calories: 70; Total Fat: 5g; Saturated Fat: 1g; Cholesterol: 0mg; Sodium: 0mg; Total Carbohydrates: 5g; Dietary Fiber: 2g; Protein: 2g

Roasted Cauliflower
INGREDIENTS:
- 1 large head cauliflower,
- 2 tablespoons olive oil,

- 1 teaspoon garlic powder

Cooking Method:
Preheat the oven to 400°F. Cut cauliflower into small florets, discarding stalks.
Place florets on a baking sheet lined with parchment paper, drizzle with olive oil, and season with garlic powder, salt, and pepper.
Bake for 20-25 minutes, stirring once halfway through.
Prep Time: 10 minutes

Nutritional Value (per serving): Calories: 70; Total Fat: 5g; Saturated Fat: 1g; Cholesterol: 0mg; Sodium: 0mg; Total Carbohydrates: 5g; Dietary Fiber: 2g; Protein: 2g

Baked Carrot Fries

INGREDIENTS:

- 2 large carrots,
- 2 tablespoons olive oil,
- 1 teaspoon garlic powder

Cooking Method:
Preheat the oven to 400°F.
Peel and cut carrots into thin strips.
Place on a baking sheet lined with parchment paper, drizzle with olive oil, and season with garlic powder, salt, and pepper.

Bake for 20-25 minutes, flipping once halfway through.
Prep Time: 10 minutes

Nutritional Value (per serving): Calories: 80; Total Fat: 5g; Saturated Fat: 1g; Cholesterol: 0mg; Sodium: 0mg; Total Carbohydrates: 8g; Dietary Fiber: 3g; Protein: 1g.

MEDITERRANEAN SOUP AND STEW RECIPES

1. Mediterranean Lentil Soup
INGREDIENTS:
- - 2 tablespoons olive oil
- - 1 large onion, diced
- - 4 cloves garlic, minced
- - 1 teaspoon cumin
- - 1 teaspoon oregano
- - ½ teaspoon black pepper
- - 2 cups vegetable broth
- - 2 cups water
- - 1 cup uncooked brown lentils
- - 2 large carrots, peeled and diced
- - 1 red bell pepper, diced
- - 1 (14.5 ounce) can diced tomatoes, drained
- - 2 tablespoons tomato paste
- - 2 tablespoons red wine vinegar
- - 1 teaspoon dried basil

Cooking Method:
1. In a large soup pot, heat the olive oil over medium heat.
2. Add the onions and garlic and sauté for 2 minutes.
3. Add the cumin, oregano, and black pepper and stir to combine.
4. Add the vegetable broth, water, lentils, carrots, bell pepper, diced tomatoes, tomato paste, red wine vinegar, and basil.
5. Bring the soup to a boil, then reduce the heat to low and simmer for 20 minutes, or until the lentils are tender.
6. Serve hot.
Prep Time: 10 minutes
Cook Time: 20 minutes

Nutritional Value (per serving):
Calories: 215
Fat: 6 g
Carbohydrates: 28 g
Protein: 11 g
Sodium: 128 mg

2. Mediterranean Chickpea Stew

INGREDIENTS:

- - 2 tablespoons olive oil
- - 1 medium onion, diced
- - 2 cloves garlic, minced
- - 1 teaspoon cumin
- - 1 teaspoon oregano
- - ½ teaspoon black pepper
- - 1 (14.5 ounce) can diced tomatoes, drained
- - 1 (15 ounce) can chickpeas, drained and rinsed
- - 2 cups vegetable broth
- - 2 tablespoons tomato paste
- - 2 tablespoons red wine vinegar
- - 1 teaspoon dried basil
- - 2 cups fresh spinach, roughly chopped

Cooking Method:
1. In a large soup pot, heat the olive oil over medium heat.
2. Add the onions and garlic and sauté for 2 minutes.
3. Add the cumin, oregano, and black pepper and stir to combine.
4. Add the diced tomatoes, chickpeas, vegetable broth, tomato paste, red wine vinegar, and basil.
5. Bring the stew to a boil, then reduce the heat to low and simmer for 15 minutes.
6. Add the spinach and simmer for an additional 5 minutes.
7. Serve hot.

Prep Time: 10 minutes
Cook Time: 20 minutes

Nutritional Value (per serving):
Calories: 160
Fat: 5 g

Carbohydrates: 24 g
Protein: 6 g
Sodium: 113 mg

3. White Bean and Kale Soup
INGREDIENTS:

- - 2 tablespoons olive oil
- - 1 large onion, diced
- - 3 cloves garlic, minced
- - 1 teaspoon cumin
- - 1 teaspoon oregano
- - ½ teaspoon black pepper
- - 2 (15 ounce) cans cannellini beans, drained and rinsed
- - 4 cups vegetable broth
- - 2 cups water
- - 1 cup uncooked brown rice
- - 2 cups kale, chopped
- - 2 tablespoons tomato paste
- - 2 tablespoons red wine vinegar
- - 1 teaspoon dried basil

Cooking Method:
1. In a large soup pot, heat the olive oil over medium heat.
2. Add the onions and garlic and sauté for 2 minutes.
3. Add the cumin, oregano, and black pepper and stir to combine.
4. Add the cannellini beans, vegetable broth, water, rice, kale, tomato paste, red wine vinegar, and basil.
5. Bring the soup to a boil, then reduce the heat to low and simmer for 20 minutes, or until the rice is cooked.
6. Serve hot.
Prep Time: 10 minutes
Cook Time: 20 minutes

Nutritional Value (per serving):
Calories: 220
Fat: 5 g
Carbohydrates: 33 g
Protein: 8 g

Sodium: 135 mg

4. Roasted Tomato and Pepper Soup

INGREDIENTS:

- - 2 tablespoons olive oil
- - 2 large tomatoes, diced
- - 1 large onion, diced
- - 2 cloves garlic, minced
- - 2 bell peppers, diced
- - 1 teaspoon cumin
- - 1 teaspoon oregano
- - ½ teaspoon black pepper
- - 4 cups vegetable broth
- - 2 tablespoons tomato paste
- - 2 tablespoons red wine vinegar
- - 1 teaspoon dried basil

Cooking Method:

1. Preheat the oven to 400°F.

2. On a large baking sheet, spread the tomatoes, onion, garlic, and bell peppers in an even layer.

3. Drizzle with the olive oil and sprinkle with the cumin, oregano, and black pepper.

4. Roast the vegetables for 25 minutes, or until lightly browned.

5. In a large soup pot, add the vegetable broth, tomato paste, red wine vinegar, and basil.

6. Add the roasted vegetables and stir to combine.

7. Bring the soup to a boil, then reduce the heat to low and simmer for 10 minutes.

8. Serve hot.

Prep Time: 10 minutes

Cook Time: 35 minutes

Nutritional Value (per serving):

Calories: 140

Fat: 5 g

Carbohydrates: 19 g
Protein: 5 g
Sodium: 132 mg

5. Greek Eggplant Stew
INGREDIENTS:
- - 2 tablespoons olive oil
- - 1 large onion, diced
- - 4 cloves garlic, minced
- - 1 teaspoon cumin
- - 1 teaspoon oregano
- - ½ teaspoon black pepper
- - 1 large eggplant, cubed
- - 2 (14.5 ounce) cans diced tomatoes, drained
- - 2 cups vegetable broth
- - 2 tablespoons tomato paste
- - 2 tablespoons red wine vinegar
- - 1 teaspoon dried basil
- - 2 tablespoons fresh parsley, chopped

Cooking Method:
1. In a large soup pot, heat the olive oil over medium heat.
2. Add the onions and garlic and sauté for 2 minutes.
3. Add the cumin, oregano, and black pepper and stir to combine.
4. Add the eggplant, diced tomatoes, vegetable broth, tomato paste, red wine vinegar, and basil.
5. Bring the stew to a boil, then reduce the heat to low and simmer for 20 minutes, or until the eggplant is tender.
6. Stir in the parsley and serve hot.
Prep Time: 10 minutes
Cook Time: 20 minutes

Nutritional Value (per serving):
Calories: 162
Fat: 5 g
Carbohydrates: 25 g
Protein: 5 g

Sodium: 127 mg

6. Greek Spinach and Feta Soup

INGREDIENTS:

- - 2 tablespoons olive oil
- - 1 large onion, diced
- - 4 cloves garlic, minced
- - 1 teaspoon cumin
- - 1 teaspoon oregano
- - ½ teaspoon black pepper
- - 2 cups vegetable broth
- - 2 cups water
- - 2 cups spinach, roughly chopped
- - 1 (14.5 ounce) can diced tomatoes, drained
- - 2 tablespoons tomato paste
- - 2 tablespoons red wine vinegar
- - 1 teaspoon dried basil
- - ½ cup crumbled feta cheese

Cooking Method:
1. In a large soup pot, heat the olive oil over medium heat.
2. Add the onions and garlic and sauté for 2 minutes.
3. Add the cumin, oregano, and black pepper and stir to combine.
4. Add the vegetable broth, water, spinach, diced tomatoes, tomato paste, red wine vinegar, and basil.
5. Bring the soup to a boil, then reduce the heat to low and simmer for 10 minutes.
6. Stir in the feta cheese and serve hot.
Prep Time: 10 minutes
Cook Time: 10 minutes

Nutritional Value (per serving):
Calories: 151
Fat: 8 g
Carbohydrates: 17 g
Protein: 5 g
Sodium: 123 mg

7. Greek Stifado (Beef Stew)

INGREDIENTS:

- - 2 tablespoons olive oil
- - 1 pound lean ground beef
- - 1 large onion, diced
- - 4 cloves garlic, minced
- - 1 teaspoon cumin
- - 1 teaspoon oregano
- - ½ teaspoon black pepper
- - 2 (14.5 ounce) cans diced tomatoes, drained
- - 2 cups vegetable broth
- - 2 tablespoons tomato paste
- - 2 tablespoons red wine vinegar
- - 1 teaspoon dried basil

Cooking Method:
1. In a large soup pot, heat the olive oil over medium heat.
2. Add the ground beef and cook until browned.
3. Add the onions and garlic and sauté for 2 minutes.
4. Add the cumin, oregano, and black pepper and stir to combine.
5. Add the diced tomatoes, vegetable broth, tomato paste, red wine vinegar, and basil.
6. Bring the stew to a boil, then reduce the heat to low and simmer for 20 minutes.
7. Serve hot.

Prep Time: 10 minutes
Cook Time: 20 minutes

Nutritional Value (per serving):
Calories: 250
Fat: 11 g

Carbohydrates: 16 g
Protein: 20 g
Sodium: 138 mg

8. Italian Minestrone Soup
INGREDIENTS:

- - 2 tablespoons olive oil
- - 1 large onion, diced
- - 4 cloves garlic, minced
- - 1 teaspoon cumin
- - 1 teaspoon oregano
- - ½ teaspoon black pepper
- - 2 (14.5 ounce) cans diced tomatoes, drained
- - 4 cups vegetable broth
- - 2 cups water
- - 1 cup uncooked small shell pasta
- - 2 cups fresh spinach, roughly chopped

- - 1 (15 ounce) can kidney beans, drained and rinsed
- - 2 tablespoons tomato paste
- - 2 tablespoons red wine vinegar
- - 1 teaspoon dried basil

Cooking Method:
1. In a large soup pot, heat the olive oil over medium heat.
2. Add the onions and garlic and sauté for 2 minutes.
3. Add the cumin, oregano, and black pepper and stir to combine.
4. Add the diced tomatoes, vegetable broth, water, shell pasta, spinach, kidney beans, tomato paste, red wine vinegar, and basil.
5. Bring the soup to a boil, then reduce the heat to low and simmer for 20 minutes, or until the pasta is cooked.
6. Serve hot.
Prep Time: 10 minutes
Cook Time: 20 minutes

Nutritional Value (per serving):
Calories: 293
Fat: 6 g
Carbohydrates: 43 g
Protein: 13 g
Sodium: 132 mg

9. Italian White Bean and Vegetable Soup

INGREDIENTS:

- - 2 tablespoons extra-virgin olive oil
- - 1 medium onion, diced
- - 2 cloves garlic, minced
- - 2 carrots, diced
- - 2 stalks celery, diced
- - 1 large potato, peeled and diced
- - 1/2 teaspoon freshly ground black pepper
- - 1 bay leaf
- - 4 cups vegetable broth

- - 2 (15-ounce) cans white beans, drained and rinsed
- - 2 cups fresh spinach, chopped
- - 2 tablespoons fresh parsley leaves, chopped
- - 2 tablespoons fresh basil leaves, chopped

Cooking Method:
1. Heat the oil in a large pot over medium heat.
2. Add the onion and garlic and cook until the onion is softened, about 5 minutes.
3. Add the carrots, celery, potato, black pepper, and bay leaf. Cook for another 5 minutes.
4. Add the vegetable broth and bring to a simmer.
5. Add the white beans and simmer for 10 minutes.
6. Add the spinach, parsley, and basil and simmer for another 5 minutes.

7. Serve hot.
Prep Time: 20 minutes

Nutritional Value: Calories: 312, Total
Fat: 6.8g, Saturated Fat: 1.1g,
Cholesterol: 0mg, Sodium: 682mg,
Carbohydrates: 45.7g, Fiber: 11.5g,
Protein: 14.6g

10. Italian Vegetable and Bean Stew
INGREDIENTS:
- - 2 tablespoons extra-virgin olive oil
- - 1 onion, diced
- - 2 cloves garlic, minced
- - 2 carrots, diced
- - 2 stalks celery, diced
- - 1 large potato, peeled and diced
- - 1/4 teaspoon freshly ground black pepper
- - 1 bay leaf

- - 2 cups vegetable broth
- - 2 (15-ounce) cans cannellini beans, drained and rinsed
- - 1/2 cup frozen green peas
- - 2 tablespoons fresh parsley leaves, chopped
- - 2 tablespoons fresh basil leaves, chopped

Cooking Method:
1. Heat the oil in a large pot over medium heat.
2. Add the onion and garlic and cook until the onion is softened, about 5 minutes.
3. Add the carrots, celery, potato, black pepper, and bay leaf. Cook for another 5 minutes.
4. Add the vegetable broth and bring to a simmer.
5. Add the cannellini beans and simmer for 10 minutes.

6. Add the green peas, parsley, and basil and simmer for another 5 minutes.
7. Serve hot.
Prep Time: 20 minutes

Nutritional Value: Calories: 327, Total Fat: 6.5g, Saturated Fat: 0.8g, Cholesterol: 0mg, Sodium: 564 mg, Carbohydrates: 49.2g, Fiber: 14.3g, Protein: 14.9g

11. Spanish Gazpacho
INGREDIENTS:
- - 2 tablespoons extra-virgin olive oil
- - 1 medium onion, diced
- - 2 cloves garlic, minced
- - 2 large tomatoes, diced
- - 1 cucumber, peeled and diced
- - 1 red bell pepper, diced
- - 1/4 teaspoon freshly ground black pepper
- - 2 cups vegetable broth

- - 2 tablespoons red wine vinegar
- - 2 tablespoons fresh parsley leaves, chopped
- - 2 tablespoons fresh basil leaves, chopped

Cooking Method:
1. Heat the oil in a large pot over medium heat.
2. Add the onion and garlic and cook until the onion is softened, about 5 minutes.
3. Add the tomatoes, cucumber, bell pepper, black pepper, and vegetable broth. Bring to a simmer.
4. Simmer for 10 minutes.
5. Add the red wine vinegar, parsley, and basil and simmer for another 5 minutes.
6. Transfer to a blender and blend until smooth.
7. Serve cold.
Prep Time: 20 minutes

Nutritional Value: Calories: 161, Total Fat: 7.1g, Saturated Fat: 1.0g, Cholesterol: 0mg, Sodium: 529 mg, Carbohydrates: 18.7g, Fiber: 5.3g, Protein: 5.3g

12. Spanish Chickpea and Spinach Stew

INGREDIENTS:

- - 2 tablespoons extra-virgin olive oil
- - 1 medium onion, diced
- - 2 cloves garlic, minced
- - 1 teaspoon paprika
- - 1/4 teaspoon freshly ground black pepper
- - 1 bay leaf
- - 2 cups vegetable broth
- - 2 (15-ounce) cans chickpeas, drained and rinsed
- - 2 cups fresh spinach, chopped

- - 2 tablespoons fresh parsley leaves, chopped
- - 2 tablespoons fresh basil leaves, chopped

Cooking Method:
1. Heat the oil in a large pot over medium heat.
2. Add the onion and garlic and cook until the onion is softened, about 5 minutes.
3. Add the paprika, black pepper, and bay leaf. Cook for another 5 minutes.
4. Add the vegetable broth and bring to a simmer.
5. Add the chickpeas and simmer for 10 minutes.
6. Add the spinach, parsley, and basil and simmer for another 5 minutes.
7. Serve hot.
Prep Time: 20 minutes

Nutritional Value: Calories: 326, Total Fat: 6.5g, Saturated Fat: 0.9g, Cholesterol: 0mg, Sodium: 589mg, Carbohydrates: 47.8g, Fiber: 12.4g, Protein: 14.8g

13. Moroccan Lentil Soup

INGREDIENTS:

- - 2 tablespoons extra-virgin olive oil
- - 1 medium onion, diced
- - 2 cloves garlic, minced
- - 1 teaspoon cumin
- - 1/2 teaspoon freshly ground black pepper
- - 1 bay leaf
- - 6 cups vegetable broth
- - 1 cup red lentils, rinsed
- - 2 tablespoons fresh parsley leaves, chopped
- - 2 tablespoons fresh cilantro leaves, chopped

Cooking Method:

1. Heat the oil in a large pot over medium heat.
2. Add the onion and garlic and cook until the onion is softened, about 5 minutes.
3. Add the cumin, black pepper, and bay leaf. Cook for another 5 minutes.
4. Add the vegetable broth and bring to a simmer.
5. Add the lentils and simmer for 15 minutes.
6. Add the parsley and cilantro and simmer for another 5 minutes.
7. Serve hot.

Prep Time: 25 minutes

Nutritional Value: Calories: 297, Total Fat: 7.3g, Saturated Fat: 1.1g, Cholesterol: 0mg, Sodium: 601mg,

Carbohydrates: 42.9g, Fiber: 13.7g,
Protein: 14.7g

14. Moroccan Chickpea and Vegetable Stew

INGREDIENTS:

- - 2 tablespoons extra-virgin olive oil
- - 1 medium onion, diced
- - 2 cloves garlic, minced
- - 1 teaspoon cumin
- - 1/2 teaspoon freshly ground black pepper
- - 1 bay leaf
- - 2 cups vegetable broth
- - 2 (15-ounce) cans chickpeas, drained and rinsed
- - 1 large potato, peeled and diced
- - 2 carrots, diced
- - 2 stalks celery, diced

- - 2 tablespoons fresh parsley leaves, chopped
- - 2 tablespoons fresh cilantro leaves, chopped

Cooking Method:
1. Heat the oil in a large pot over medium heat.
2. Add the onion and garlic and cook until the onion is softened, about 5 minutes.
3. Add the cumin, black pepper, and bay leaf. Cook for another 5 minutes.
4. Add the vegetable broth, chickpeas, potato, carrots, and celery. Bring to a simmer.
5. Simmer for 10 minutes.
6. Add the parsley and cilantro and simmer for another 5 minutes.
7. Serve hot.

Prep Time: 20 minutes

Nutritional Value: Calories: 335, Total Fat: 6.5g, Saturated Fat: 0.9g, Cholesterol: 0mg, Sodium: 583mg, Carbohydrates: 52.6g, Fiber: 13.2g, Protein: 15.9g

15. Turkish Red Lentil Soup
INGREDIENTS:
- - 2 tablespoons extra-virgin olive oil
- - 1 medium onion, diced
- - 2 cloves garlic, minced
- - 1 teaspoon cumin
- - 1/2 teaspoon freshly ground black pepper
- - 1 bay leaf
- - 6 cups vegetable broth
- - 1 cup red lentils, rinsed
- - 1/4 cup tomato paste
- - 2 tablespoons fresh parsley leaves, chopped

- - 2 tablespoons fresh dill leaves, chopped

Cooking Method:
1. Heat the oil in a large pot over medium heat.
2. Add the onion and garlic and cook until the onion is softened, about 5 minutes.
3. Add the cumin, black pepper, and bay leaf. Cook for another 5 minutes.
4. Add the vegetable broth and bring to a simmer.
5. Add the lentils and tomato paste and simmer for 15 minutes.
6. Add the parsley and dill and simmer for another 5 minutes.
7. Serve hot.
Prep Time: 20 minutes

Nutritional Value: Calories: 296, Total Fat: 7.2g, Saturated Fat: 1.1g, Cholesterol: 0mg, Sodium: 656 mg,

Carbohydrates: 42.5g, Fiber: 14.7g,
Protein: 14.5g

CHAPTER 5: HIGH BLOOD PRESSURE LOWERING SEAFOOD AND POULTRY MAINS RECIPES

1. Grilled Salmon with Herbs

INGREDIENTS:

- 4 (6-ounce) Salmon Filets
- 2 tablespoons Olive Oil
- Freshly Ground Black Pepper
- 2 tablespoons Chopped Fresh Herbs (such as Parsley, Basil, and Oregano)

Prep Time: 10 minutes
Cook Time: 10 minutes

Cooking method:
1. Preheat a grill to medium-high heat.

2. Rub the salmon filets with the olive oil and season with black pepper.
3. Place the salmon on the preheated grill and cook for 4 minutes. Flip the salmon and cook for an additional 4 minutes or until the salmon is cooked through.
4. Remove the salmon from the grill and top with the chopped herbs.

Nutrition:
Calories: 336 kcal, Carbohydrates: 0.5 g, Protein: 40 g, Fat: 18.5 g, Saturated Fat: 2.5 g, Cholesterol: 97 mg, Sodium: 67 mg, Fiber: 0.2 g, Sugar: 0 g.

2. Baked Tilapia with Lemon
INGREDIENTS:
- 4 (4-ounce) Tilapia Filets
- 2 tablespoons Olive Oil
- Freshly Ground Black Pepper
- 2 tablespoons Lemon Juice

- 2 tablespoons Chopped Fresh Parsley

Prep Time: 10 minutes
Cook Time: 20 minutes

Cooking method:
1. Preheat the oven to 350°F (175°C).
2. Rub the tilapia filets with the olive oil and season with black pepper.
3. Place the filets on a baking sheet and bake in the preheated oven for 20 minutes.
4. Remove the tilapia from the oven and top with the lemon juice and parsley.

Nutrition:
Calories: 224 kcal, Carbohydrates: 0.5 g, Protein: 30 g, Fat: 10 g, Saturated Fat: 1.5 g, Cholesterol: 56 mg, Sodium: 66 mg, Fiber: 0.2 g, Sugar: 0 g.

3. Roasted Lemon-Garlic Chicken

INGREDIENTS:

- 4 (4-ounce) Chicken Breasts
- 2 tablespoons Olive Oil
- Freshly Ground Black Pepper
- 2 cloves Garlic, minced
- 2 tablespoons Lemon Juice
- 2 tablespoons Chopped Fresh Parsley

Prep Time: 10 minutes
Cook Time: 20 minutes

Cooking method:
1. Preheat the oven to 350°F (175°C).
2. Rub the chicken breasts with the olive oil and season with black pepper.
3. Place the chicken on a baking sheet and bake in the preheated oven for 20 minutes.

4. Remove the chicken from the oven and top with the garlic, lemon juice, and parsley.

Nutrition:
Calories: 246 kcal, Carbohydrates: 0.5 g, Protein: 32 g, Fat: 11 g, Saturated Fat: 1.5 g, Cholesterol: 82 mg, Sodium: 79 mg, Fiber: 0.2 g, Sugar: 0 g.

4. Poached Cod with White Wine
INGREDIENTS:
- 4 (4-ounce) Cod Filets
- 2 tablespoons Olive Oil
- Freshly Ground Black Pepper
- 1 cup White Wine
- 2 tablespoons Chopped Fresh Parsley

Prep Time: 10 minutes
Cook Time: 15 minutes

Cooking method:
1. Heat a large skillet over medium-high heat and add the olive oil.
2. Season the cod filets with black pepper and add to the skillet.
3. Add the white wine to the skillet and bring to a boil.
4. Reduce the heat to low and simmer for 15 minutes or until the cod is cooked through.
5. Remove the cod from the skillet and top with the chopped parsley.

Nutrition:
Calories: 246 kcal, Carbohydrates: 0.5 g, Protein: 32 g, Fat: 11 g, Saturated Fat: 1.5 g, Cholesterol: 82 mg, Sodium: 79 mg, Fiber: 0.2 g, Sugar: 0 g.

5. Grilled Halibut with Citrus Salsa
INGREDIENTS:
- 4 (4-ounce) Halibut Filets
- 2 tablespoons Olive Oil
- Freshly Ground Black Pepper
- 2 tablespoons Chopped Fresh Cilantro
- 2 tablespoons Chopped Fresh Parsley
- 2 tablespoons Chopped Fresh Mint
- 1/2 cup Orange Juice
- 1/2 cup Lime Juice

Prep Time: 10 minutes
Cook Time: 10 minutes

Cooking method:
1. Preheat a grill to medium-high heat.
2. Rub the halibut filets with the olive oil and season with black pepper.
3. Place the halibut on the preheated grill and cook for 4 minutes. Flip the halibut

and cook for an additional 4 minutes or until the halibut is cooked through.

4. Remove the halibut from the grill and top with the cilantro, parsley, mint, orange juice, and lime juice.

Nutrition:
Calories: 304 kcal, Carbohydrates: 6.5 g, Protein: 34 g, Fat: 15 g, Saturated Fat: 2.5 g, Cholesterol: 82 mg, Sodium: 77 mg, Fiber: 1.3 g, Sugar: 2.3 g.

6. Baked Salmon with Basil
INGREDIENTS:
- 4 (6-ounce) Salmon Filets
- 2 tablespoons Olive Oil
- Freshly Ground Black Pepper
- 2 tablespoons Chopped Fresh Basil

Prep Time: 10 minutes
Cook Time: 10 minutes

Cooking method:
1. Preheat the oven to 350°F (175°C).
2. Rub the salmon filets with the olive oil and season with black pepper.
3. Place the salmon on a baking sheet and bake in the preheated oven for 10 minutes.
4. Remove the salmon from the oven and top with the chopped basil.

Nutrition:
Calories: 336 kcal, Carbohydrates: 0.5 g, Protein: 40 g, Fat: 18.5 g, Saturated Fat: 2.5 g, Cholesterol: 97 mg, Sodium: 67 mg, Fiber: 0.2 g, Sugar: 0 g.

7. Steamed Shrimp with Garlic
INGREDIENTS:
- 1 pound Raw Shrimp, peeled and deveined

- 2 tablespoons Olive Oil
- Freshly Ground Black Pepper
- 2 cloves Garlic, minced
- 2 tablespoons Chopped Fresh Parsley

Prep Time: 10 minutes
Cook Time: 8 minutes

Instructions:
1. Fill a large pot with an inch of water and place a steamer insert inside. Bring the water to a boil.
2. Rub the shrimp with the olive oil and season with black pepper.
3. Place the shrimp in the steamer insert and cover. Steam for 8 minutes or until the shrimp are cooked through.
4. Remove the shrimp from the steamer and top with the garlic and parsley.

Nutrition:

Calories: 236 kcal, Carbohydrates: 0.5 g,
Protein: 34 g, Fat: 10 g, Saturated Fat: 1.5
g, Cholesterol: 288 mg, Sodium: 241 mg,
Fiber: 0.2 g, Sugar: 0 g.

8. Broiled Scallops with Parsley
INGREDIENTS:
- 1 pound Sea Scallops
- 2 tablespoons Olive Oil
- Freshly Ground Black Pepper
- 2 tablespoons Chopped Fresh Parsley

Prep Time: 10 minutes
Cook Time: 8 minutes

Cooking method:
1. Preheat the oven to broil.
2. Rub the scallops with the olive oil and season with black pepper.

3. Place the scallops on a baking sheet and broil in the preheated oven for 8 minutes or until the scallops are cooked through.
4. Remove the scallops from the oven and top with the chopped parsley.

Nutrition:
Calories: 216 kcal, Carbohydrates: 0.5 g, Protein: 35 g, Fat: 8 g, Saturated Fat: 1 g, Cholesterol: 54 mg, Sodium: 80 mg, Fiber: 0.2 g, Sugar: 0 g.

9. Grilled Shrimp with Tomato-Olive Relish
INGREDIENTS:
- 1 pound Raw Shrimp, peeled and deveined
- 2 tablespoons Olive Oil
- Freshly Ground Black Pepper
- 1/2 cup Chopped Tomatoes

- 1/2 cup Chopped Olives
- 2 tablespoons Chopped Fresh Parsley

Prep Time: 10 minutes
Cook Time: 8 minutes

Cooking method:
1. Preheat a grill to medium-high heat.
2. Rub the shrimp with the olive oil and season with black pepper.
3. Place the shrimp on the preheated grill and cook for 4 minutes. Flip the shrimp and cook for an additional 4 minutes or until the shrimp are cooked through.
4. Remove the shrimp from the grill and top with the tomatoes, olives, and parsley.

Nutrition:
Calories: 236 kcal, Carbohydrates: 4 g, Protein: 34 g, Fat: 10 g, Saturated Fat: 1.5

g, Cholesterol: 288 mg, Sodium: 241 mg, Fiber: 1.1 g, Sugar: 1.3 g.

10. Baked Sea Bass with Dill

INGREDIENTS:

- 4 (4-ounce) Sea Bass Filets
- 2 tablespoons Olive Oil
- Freshly Ground Black Pepper
- 2 tablespoons Chopped Fresh Dill

Prep Time: 10 minutes
Cook Time: 15 minutes

Cooking method:
1. Preheat the oven to 350°F (175°C).
2. Rub the sea bass filets with the olive oil and season with black pepper.
3. Place the filets on a baking sheet and bake in the preheated oven for 15 minutes.

4. Remove the sea bass from the oven and top with the chopped dill.

Nutrition:
Calories: 212 kcal, Carbohydrates: 0.3 g, Protein: 33 g, Fat: 8 g, Saturated Fat: 1 g, Cholesterol: 56 mg, Sodium: 74 mg, Fiber: 0.1 g, Sugar: 0 g.

11. Grilled Trout with Lemon Butter
INGREDIENTS:
- - 2 (6 ounce) trout filets
- - 2 tablespoons butter
- - 2 tablespoons lemon juice
- - 2 tablespoons fresh parsley, chopped

Cooking method:
1. Preheat the grill to medium heat.
2. Place trout filets on the grill and cook for 3 to 5 minutes.

3. Flip the trout over and cook for an additional 3 to 5 minutes.

4. Meanwhile, melt the butter in a small saucepan over low heat.

5. Add the lemon juice and parsley, stirring to combine.

6. Remove the trout from the grill and spoon the lemon butter over the top.

Prep time: 10 minutes
Nutritional value: Calories: 244; Protein: 22.9g; Fat: 14.7g; Carbs: 1.1g; Sodium: 69mg; Fiber: 0.4g

12. Poached Cod with Spinach
INGREDIENTS:
- - 2 (6 ounce) fresh cod filets
- - 1/2 cup white wine
- - 2 tablespoons olive oil
- - 2 cups fresh spinach

Cooking method:
1. Heat olive oil in a large skillet over medium heat.
2. Add cod filets to the skillet and cook for 2 to 3 minutes.
3. Carefully pour the white wine into the skillet, cover, and reduce heat to low.
4. Simmer for 8 to 10 minutes, or until the fish flakes easily with a fork.
5. Add the spinach to the skillet and cook for an additional 3 to 4 minutes, or until the spinach is wilted.

Prep time: 15 minutes
Nutritional value: Calories: 278; Protein: 34.4g; Fat: 11.2g; Carbs: 2.4g; Sodium: 57mg; Fiber: 1.7g

13. Roasted Turkey Breast with Herbs

INGREDIENTS:

- - 2 (6 ounce) boneless, skinless turkey breasts
- - 2 tablespoons olive oil
- - 1 teaspoon fresh thyme, chopped
- - 1 teaspoon fresh rosemary, chopped
- - 1/2 teaspoon garlic powder

Cooking method:

1. Preheat the oven to 375 degrees F (190 degrees C).
2. Place turkey breasts side by side in a shallow baking dish.
3. Drizzle olive oil over the breasts and season with thyme, rosemary, and garlic powder.
4. Bake in a preheated oven for 25 to 30 minutes, or until the internal temperature of the turkey breasts reaches 165 degrees F (75 degrees C).

Prep time: 10 minutes
Nutritional value: Calories: 286; Protein: 35.3g; Fat: 13.3g; Carbs: 0.3g; Sodium: 121mg; Fiber: 0.2g

14. Baked Halibut with Olive Tapenade

INGREDIENTS:

- - 2 (6 ounce) halibut filets
- - 2 tablespoons olive tapenade
- - 2 tablespoons white wine
- - 1 tablespoon freshly squeezed lemon juice

Cooking method:

1. Preheat the oven to 375 degrees F (190 degrees C).
2. Place halibut filets in a shallow baking dish.

3. Spread olive tapenade over the top of the filets and pour white wine and lemon juice around the filets.

4. Bake in a preheated oven for 15 to 20 minutes, or until the fish flakes easily with a fork.

Prep time: 10 minutes
Nutritional value: Calories: 224; Protein: 32.4g; Fat: 6.6g; Carbs: 2.9g; Sodium: 145mg; Fiber: 0.6g

15. Steamed Mussels with Garlic
INGREDIENTS:
- - 2 pounds fresh mussels
- - 2 tablespoons olive oil
- - 2 cloves garlic, minced
- - 1/4 cup white wine
- - 2 tablespoons freshly squeezed lemon juice

Cooking method:
1. Heat olive oil in a large pot over medium heat.
2. Add garlic and cook for 1 minute, stirring frequently.
3. Add mussels, white wine, and lemon juice to the pot.
4. Cover and steam for 8 to 10 minutes, or until the mussels have opened.

Prep time: 10 minutes
Nutritional value: Calories: 281; Protein: 32.4g; Fat: 11.2g; Carbs: 5.7g; Sodium: 139 mg; Fiber: 0.3g

16. Broiled Tilapia with Pesto
INGREDIENTS:
- - 2 (6 ounce) tilapia filets
- - 2 tablespoons pesto
- - 2 tablespoons olive oil

Cooking method:
1. Preheat the broiler.
2. Place tilapia filets on a greased broiling pan.
3. Spread pesto over the top of the filets and drizzle with olive oil.
4. Broil for 8 to 10 minutes, or until the fish flakes easily with a fork.

Prep time: 10 minutes
Nutritional value: Calories: 289; Protein: 32.8g; Fat: 14.6g; Carbs: 2.2g; Sodium: 205 mg; Fiber: 0.9g

17. Grilled Salmon with Mango Salsa

INGREDIENTS:
- - 2 (6 ounce) salmon filets
- - 2 tablespoons olive oil
- - 1 cup mango salsa

Cooking method:
1. Preheat the grill to medium heat.
2. Brush salmon filets with olive oil and place on the preheated grill.
3. Grill for 6 to 8 minutes, or until the fish flakes easily with a fork.
4. Serve with mango salsa.

Prep time: 10 minutes
Nutritional value: Calories: 292; Protein: 31.4g; Fat: 13.9g; Carbs: 9.7g; Sodium: 56mg; Fiber: 1.8g

18. Baked Trout with Dill
INGREDIENTS:
- - 2 (6 ounce) trout filets
- - 2 tablespoons olive oil
- - 1 tablespoon fresh dill, chopped
- - 2 tablespoons freshly squeezed lemon juice

Cooking method:

1. Preheat the oven to 375 degrees F (190 degrees C).

2. Place trout filets in a shallow baking dish.

3. Drizzle olive oil over the top of the filets and sprinkle with dill and lemon juice.

4. Bake in a preheated oven for 15 to 20 minutes, or until the fish flakes easily with a fork.

Prep time: 10 minutes

Nutritional value: Calories: 259; Protein: 27.4g; Fat: 12.3g; Carbs: 1.9g; Sodium: 79 mg; Fiber: 0.8g

19. Roasted Chicken Breast with Rosemary

INGREDIENTS:

- 4 chicken breasts,
- 1 tablespoon of olive oil,

- 1 tablespoon of fresh rosemary,
- 1 tablespoon of freshly ground black pepper

Cooking Method:
1. Preheat the oven to 375°F.
2. Place chicken breasts in an oven-safe dish.
3. Drizzle olive oil over chicken and sprinkle with rosemary and black pepper.
4. Bake chicken in a preheated oven for 30-40 minutes, or until cooked through.

Prep Time: 10 minutes
Cook Time: 40 minutes
Nutritional Value: calories: 285, fat: 12g, protein: 40g, carbohydrates: 0g

20. Poached Salmon with Mustard Sauce

INGREDIENTS:

- 4 salmon filets,
- 1 tablespoon of olive oil,
- 1 tablespoon of dijon mustard,
- 1 tablespoon of honey

Cooking Method:

1. Heat a pot of water to a low simmer.
2. Place salmon filets in the simmering water and cook for 8-10 minutes, or until cooked through.
3. Remove salmon from the pot and set aside.
4. In a small bowl, whisk together olive oil, dijon mustard, and honey.
5. Drizzle mustard sauce over cooked salmon and serve.

Prep Time: 10 minutes
Cook Time: 10 minutes

Nutritional Value: calories: 224, fat: 8g, protein: 31g, carbohydrates: 3g

21. Grilled Tuna with Ginger-Cilantro Sauce
INGREDIENTS:
- 4 tuna steaks,
- 1 tablespoon of olive oil,
- 1 tablespoon of freshly grated ginger,
- 1 tablespoon of fresh cilantro

Cooking Method:
1. Heat a grill to medium-high heat.
2. Brush tuna steaks with olive oil and season with freshly grated ginger.
3. Place tuna steaks on the grill and cook for 3-4 minutes per side, or until cooked through.
4. Remove tuna steaks from the grill and set aside.

5. In a small bowl, mix together cilantro and olive oil to form a sauce.
6. Drizzle cilantro sauce over cooked tuna and serve.

Prep Time: 10 minutes
Cook Time: 10 minutes
Nutritional Value: calories: 170, fat: 5g, protein: 30g, carbohydrates: 0g

22. Baked Halibut with Tomato-Basil Topping

INGREDIENTS:
- 4 halibut filets,
- 1 tablespoon of olive oil,
- 1 tablespoon of diced tomatoes,
- 1 tablespoon of chopped fresh basil

Cooking Method:
1. Preheat the oven to 375°F.

2. Place halibut filets in an oven-safe dish.

3. Drizzle olive oil over the halibut and season with salt and pepper.

4. Bake in a preheated oven for 15-20 minutes, or until cooked through.

5. Remove halibut from the oven and top with diced tomatoes and chopped basil.

6. Return to the oven and bake for an additional 5 minutes.

Prep Time: 10 minutes
Cook Time: 25 minutes
Nutritional Value: calories: 201, fat: 7g, protein: 30g, carbohydrates: 2g

23. Steamed Clams with Garlic and Herbs

INGREDIENTS:
- 2 dozen clams,
- 1 tablespoon of olive oil,

- 1 tablespoon of minced garlic,
- 1 tablespoon of chopped fresh herbs (thyme, oregano, parsley)

Cooking Method:
1. Heat a pot of water to a low simmer.
2. Place clams in the water and cook for 8-10 minutes, or until clams open.
3. Remove clams from the pot and set aside.
4. In a small bowl, mix together olive oil, garlic, and herbs to form a sauce.
5. Drizzle sauce over cooked clams and serve.

Prep Time: 10 minutes
Cook Time: 10 minutes
Nutritional Value: calories: 28, fat: 1g, protein: 4g, carbohydrates: 0g

24. Broiled Salmon with Mango Salsa

INGREDIENTS:

- 4 salmon filets,
- 1 tablespoon of olive oil,
- 1 tablespoon of diced mango,
- 1 tablespoon of diced red onion

Cooking Method:

1. Preheat the oven to broil.
2. Place salmon filets in a baking dish.
3. Drizzle olive oil over salmon and season with salt and pepper.
4. Broil salmon in a preheated oven for 10-12 minutes, or until cooked through.
5. Remove salmon from the oven and top with mango and red onion.
6. Return to the oven and broil for an additional 5 minutes.

Prep Time: 10 minutes
Cook Time: 17 minutes

Nutritional Value: calories: 248, fat: 10g, protein: 32g, carbohydrates: 5g

25. Roasted Turkey with Parsley and Sage

INGREDIENTS:

- 1 pound of ground turkey,
- 1 tablespoon of olive oil,
- 1 tablespoon of chopped fresh parsley,
- 1 tablespoon of chopped fresh sage

Cooking Method:

1. Preheat the oven to 375°F.
2. Place ground turkey in an oven-safe dish.
3. Drizzle olive oil over turkey and season with salt and pepper.
4. Bake in a preheated oven for 20-30 minutes, or until cooked through.

5. Remove turkey from the oven and top with parsley and sage.
6. Return to the oven and bake for an additional 5 minutes.

Prep Time: 10 minutes
Cook Time: 35 minutes
Nutritional Value: calories: 209, fat: 10g, protein: 28g, carbohydrates: 0g

BEEF AND PORK MAINS

1. Slow Cooker Korean Beef Short Ribs

INGREDIENTS:

- - 4 lbs beef short ribs
- - 1/4 cup low-sodium soy sauce
- - 2 tablespoons fresh grated ginger
- - 1 tablespoon sesame oil
- - 2 garlic cloves, minced
- - 1/4 cup honey
- - 2 tablespoons rice vinegar
- - 2 tablespoons toasted sesame seeds
- - 2 scallions, chopped

Cooking Method:

1. Place the beef short ribs in the slow cooker.
2. In a medium bowl, whisk together the soy sauce, ginger, sesame oil, garlic, honey, and rice vinegar.

3. Pour the mixture over the short ribs and stir to combine.

4. Cover and cook on low for 8-10 hours.

5. Once the short ribs are cooked, remove them from the slow cooker, and transfer to a serving platter.

6. Garnish with sesame seeds, scallions, and serve.

Prep Time: 10 minutes
Cook Time: 8-10 hours
Nutritional Value: Calories: 575, Fat: 23 g, Carbohydrates: 19 g, Protein: 57 g

2. Balsamic Glazed Pork Chops

INGREDIENTS:

- - 4 (4-ounce) boneless pork chops
- - 1/4 cup balsamic vinegar
- - 2 tablespoons honey
- - 1 tablespoon Dijon mustard
- - 1/4 teaspoon freshly ground black pepper

Cooking Method:
1. Preheat the oven to 375°F.
2. Place pork chops in an oven-safe baking dish.
3. In a small bowl, whisk together the balsamic vinegar, honey, Dijon mustard, and pepper.
4. Pour the glaze over the pork chops.
5. Bake for 20 minutes, or until pork chops are cooked through.

Prep Time: 10 minutes
Cook Time: 20 minutes
Nutritional Value: Calories: 218, Fat: 8 g, Carbohydrates: 8 g, Protein: 28 g

3. Roast Pork Tenderloin with Apple-Cranberry Compote
INGREDIENTS:
- - 1 (1-pound) pork tenderloin

- - 1/2 teaspoon freshly ground black pepper
- - 1 tablespoon olive oil
- - 1/2 cup diced apples
- - 1/2 cup dried cranberries
- - 2 tablespoons honey
- - 2 tablespoons apple cider vinegar

Cooking Method:
1. Preheat the oven to 350°F.
2. Rub the pork tenderloin with pepper and olive oil.
3. Place the pork tenderloin in a roasting pan and roast for 25 minutes.
4. Meanwhile, in a medium saucepan, combine the apples, cranberries, honey, and apple cider vinegar. Cook over medium heat for 5 minutes.
5. Once the pork tenderloin is cooked, remove it from the oven and let it rest for 5 minutes before slicing.
6. Serve the pork tenderloin with the apple-cranberry compote.

Prep Time: 10 minutes
Cook Time: 30 minutes
Nutritional Value: Calories: 311, Fat: 8 g,
Carbohydrates: 25 g, Protein: 32 g

4. Pork and Apricot Meatballs

INGREDIENTS:

- - 1 lb ground pork
- - 1/4 cup diced dried apricots
- - 1/4 cup diced onion
- - 1/4 cup panko breadcrumbs
- - 1 large egg, lightly beaten
- - 2 tablespoons olive oil
- - 1/4 teaspoon ground cinnamon

Cooking Method:

1. Preheat the oven to 375°F.
2. In a large bowl, combine the ground
pork, dried apricots, onion, panko
breadcrumbs, egg, and cinnamon.

3. Use your hands to mix the INGREDIENTS until fully combined.

4. Form the mixture into small meatballs, about 2 inches in diameter.

5. Place the meatballs on a baking sheet lined with parchment paper.

6. Drizzle the olive oil over the meatballs and bake for 20 minutes, or until cooked through.

Prep Time: 10 minutes
Cook Time: 20 minutes
Nutritional Value: Calories: 212, Fat: 11 g, Carbohydrates: 8 g, Protein: 19 g

5. Slow Cooker Pulled Pork with Apple Slaw

INGREDIENTS:

- - 4 lb pork shoulder
- - 1 teaspoon freshly ground black pepper

- - 1/4 cup apple cider vinegar
- - 1/4 cup honey
- - 1/4 cup low-sodium soy sauce
- - 2 tablespoons olive oil
- - 1/2 head cabbage, thinly sliced
- - 1 large apple, cored and diced
- - 2 tablespoons Dijon mustard

Cooking Method:
1. Place the pork shoulder in the slow cooker and season with pepper.
2. In a medium bowl, whisk together the apple cider vinegar, honey, soy sauce, and olive oil.
3. Pour the mixture over the pork shoulder and stir to combine.
4. Cover and cook on low for 8-10 hours.
5. Once the pork is cooked, remove it from the slow cooker and shred with two forks.
6. In a large bowl, combine the cabbage and apple.

7. Add the shredded pork and Dijon mustard to the cabbage and apple mixture and stir to combine.

Prep Time: 10 minutes
Cook Time: 8-10 hours
Nutritional Value: Calories: 406, Fat: 20 g, Carbohydrates: 19 g, Protein: 38 g

6. Lime-Garlic Pork Tenderloin with Grilled Pineapple
INGREDIENTS:
- - 2 (1-pound) pork tenderloins
- - 2 tablespoons olive oil
- - 2 tablespoons freshly squeezed lime juice
- - 2 garlic cloves, minced
- - 1/2 teaspoon freshly ground black pepper
- - 1/4 teaspoon ground cumin
- - 2 cups pineapple chunks

Cooking Method:
1. Preheat the oven to 375°F.
2. Place the pork tenderloins in a roasting pan.
3. In a small bowl, whisk together the olive oil, lime juice, garlic, pepper, and cumin.
4. Pour the mixture over the pork tenderloins and rub to coat.
5. Roast for 25 minutes, or until pork is cooked through.
6. Meanwhile, heat a grill pan over medium-high heat.
7. Add the pineapple chunks and cook for 5 minutes, or until lightly charred.
8. Serve the pork tenderloins with the grilled pineapple.

Prep Time: 10 minutes
Cook Time: 30 minutes
Nutritional Value: Calories: 341, Fat: 8 g, Carbohydrates: 35 g, Protein: 33 g

7. Baked Pork and Apple Empanadas

INGREDIENTS:

- - 1 lb ground pork
- - 1 teaspoon freshly ground black pepper
- - 1/2 teaspoon ground cumin
- - 1/2 teaspoon garlic powder
- - 1/2 teaspoon onion powder
- - 1/2 cup diced apples
- - 2 tablespoons honey
- - 1 package (14.1-ounce) empanada discs

Cooking Method:

1. Preheat the oven to 375°F.
2. In a large bowl, combine the ground pork, pepper, cumin, garlic powder, onion powder, apples, and honey.
3. Use your hands to mix the INGREDIENTS until fully combined.

4. Place 1 tablespoon of the pork mixture onto each empanada disc.

5. Fold the empanada disc in half and press to seal the edges.

6. Place the empanadas on a baking sheet lined with parchment paper.

7. Bake for 15-20 minutes, or until golden brown.

Prep Time: 10 minutes
Cook Time: 15-20 minutes
Nutritional Value: Calories: 125, Fat: 4 g, Carbohydrates: 14 g, Protein: 8 g

8. Pork and Butternut Squash Stew

INGREDIENTS:

- - 1 tablespoon olive oil
- - 2 pounds pork shoulder, cubed
- - 1 onion, diced
- - 2 cloves garlic, minced
- - 2 cups chicken broth

- - 1 teaspoon dried oregano
- - 1 teaspoon ground cumin
- - 1 teaspoon smoked paprika
- - 2 cups cubed butternut squash
- - 1/2 teaspoon freshly ground black pepper

Cooking Method:

1. Heat the oil in a large pot over medium heat.
2. Add the pork shoulder cubes and cook until browned, about 5 minutes.
3. Add the onion and garlic and cook for another 5 minutes.
4. Add the chicken broth, oregano, cumin, and smoked paprika and bring to a simmer.
5. Add the butternut squash and black pepper and simmer for 25 minutes, stirring occasionally.
6. Serve hot.

Prep Time: 30 minutes

Nutritional Value: Calories: 283, Fat: 13g, Saturated fat: 3.6g, Carbohydrates: 11.5g, Protein: 24.2g

9. Pork Schnitzel with Lemon-Caper Sauce
INGREDIENTS:
- - 2 pounds boneless pork chops, pounded thin
- - 1 cup all-purpose flour
- - 2 eggs, beaten
- - 2 cups panko breadcrumbs
- - 1 teaspoon freshly ground black pepper
- - 1 teaspoon dried oregano
- - 1/4 cup olive oil
- - 2 tablespoons capers
- - 2 tablespoons freshly squeezed lemon juice

Cooking Method:
1. Place the flour, eggs, and panko breadcrumbs in three separate shallow bowls.
2. Season the pork chops with the pepper and oregano and dredge them in the flour, then dip them in the eggs, and finally coat them with the panko crumbs.
3. Heat the olive oil in a large skillet over medium-high heat.
4. Add the pork chops and cook until golden brown, about 3 minutes per side.
5. Transfer the pork chops to a plate and keep warm.
6. Reduce the heat to low and add the capers and lemon juice to the skillet. Simmer for 3 minutes.
7. Pour the sauce over the pork chops and serve.

Prep Time: 30 minutes

Nutritional Value: Calories: 603, Fat: 28.4g, Saturated fat: 5.8g, Carbohydrates: 34.9g, Protein: 47.8g

10. Braised Pork Ragu with Fennel

INGREDIENTS:

- - 2 tablespoons olive oil
- - 2 pounds boneless pork shoulder, cubed
- - 1 onion, diced
- - 2 cloves garlic, minced
- - 2 cups chicken broth
- - 1 teaspoon dried oregano
- - 1 teaspoon ground cumin
- - 1 teaspoon smoked paprika
- - 1 fennel bulb, thinly sliced
- - 2 tablespoons tomato paste
- - 1/2 teaspoon freshly ground black pepper

Cooking Method:
1. Heat the oil in a large pot over medium heat.
2. Add the pork shoulder cubes and cook until browned, about 5 minutes.
3. Add the onion and garlic and cook for another 5 minutes.
4. Add the chicken broth, oregano, cumin, and smoked paprika and bring to a simmer.
5. Add the fennel, tomato paste, and black pepper and simmer for 25 minutes, stirring occasionally.
6. Serve hot.

Prep Time: 30 minutes

Nutritional Value: Calories: 393, Fat: 19.2g, Saturated fat: 5.3g, Carbohydrates: 13.6g, Protein: 38.4g

11. Grilled Pork Chops with Peach Salsa

INGREDIENTS:

- - 2 tablespoons olive oil
- - 2 tablespoons freshly squeezed lime juice
- - 2 cloves garlic, minced
- - 2 teaspoons ground cumin
- - 2 teaspoons smoked paprika
- - 4 (6-ounce) boneless pork chops
- - 1/2 teaspoon freshly ground black pepper
- - 1/2 teaspoon salt
- - 1 peach, peeled and diced
- - 1/4 cup chopped fresh cilantro
- - 2 tablespoons diced red onion

Cooking Method:

1. In a small bowl, mix together the olive oil, lime juice, garlic, cumin, and smoked paprika.

2. Rub the mixture onto the pork chops and season with pepper and salt.

3. Heat a grill or grill pan over medium-high heat.

4. Add the pork chops and cook for 4 minutes per side or until cooked through.

5. Meanwhile, in a medium bowl, mix together the peach, cilantro, and red onion.

6. Serve the pork chops topped with the peach salsa.

Prep Time: 15 minutes

Nutritional Value: Calories: 415, Fat: 20.2g, Saturated fat: 5.7g, Carbohydrates: 8.9g, Protein: 44.7g

12. Spicy Pork and Sweet Potato Stir-Fry
INGREDIENTS:

- - 2 tablespoons sesame oil
- - 2 tablespoons soy sauce
- - 2 tablespoons freshly squeezed lime juice
- - 2 cloves garlic, minced
- - 1 teaspoon finely grated ginger
- - 1 teaspoon crushed red pepper flakes
- - 2 tablespoons olive oil
- - 1 pound pork tenderloin, cut into thin strips
- - 1 sweet potato, peeled and cut into thin strips
- - 1 red bell pepper, seeded and diced
- - 2 green onions, chopped
- - 1/2 teaspoon freshly ground black pepper

Cooking Method:

1. In a small bowl, mix together the sesame oil, soy sauce, lime juice, garlic, ginger, and red pepper flakes.
2. Heat the olive oil in a large skillet over medium-high heat.
3. Add the pork strips and sweet potato and cook for 5 minutes, stirring occasionally.
4. Add the bell pepper and green onions and cook for another 5 minutes.
5. Add the sesame oil mixture and black pepper and cook for 1 more minute.
6. Serve hot.

Prep Time: 15 minutes

Nutritional Value: Calories: 397, Fat: 23.2g, Saturated fat: 4.5g, Carbohydrates: 16.7g, Protein: 32.2g

13. Tequila-Lime Marinated Pork Tenderloin

INGREDIENTS:

- - 2 tablespoons tequila
- - 2 tablespoons freshly squeezed lime juice
- - 1 tablespoon olive oil
- - 1 teaspoon dried oregano
- - 1 teaspoon ground cumin
- - 1 teaspoon smoked paprika
- - 2 cloves garlic, minced
- - 1 pound pork tenderloin
- - 1/2 teaspoon freshly ground black pepper

Cooking Method:
1. In a small bowl, mix together the tequila, lime juice, olive oil, oregano, cumin, smoked paprika, and garlic.
2. Place the pork tenderloin in a shallow dish and pour the marinade over it.

3. Cover and refrigerate for at least 1 hour.

4. Preheat the grill or grill pan to medium-high heat.

5. Remove the pork from the marinade and season with the black pepper.

6. Grill the pork for 10 minutes per side or until cooked through.

7. Serve hot.

Prep Time: 1 hour and 10 minutes

Nutritional Value: Calories: 225, Fat: 10.1g, Saturated fat: 2.6g, Carbohydrates: 1.7g, Protein: 28.6g

14. Grilled Pork Chops with Mango Salsa

INGREDIENTS:
- - 2 tablespoons olive oil

- - 2 tablespoons freshly squeezed lime juice
- - 2 cloves garlic, minced
- - 2 teaspoons ground cumin
- - 2 teaspoons smoked paprika
- - 4 (6-ounce) boneless pork chops
- - 1/2 teaspoon freshly ground black pepper
- - 1/2 teaspoon salt
- - 1 mango, peeled and diced
- - 1/4 cup chopped fresh cilantro
- - 2 tablespoons diced red onion

Cooking Method:
1. In a small bowl, mix together the olive oil, lime juice, garlic, cumin, and smoked paprika.
2. Rub the mixture onto the pork chops and season with pepper and salt.
3. Heat a grill or grill pan over medium-high heat.

4. Add the pork chops and cook for 4 minutes per side or until cooked through.
5. Meanwhile, in a medium bowl, mix together the mango, cilantro, and red onion.
6. Serve the pork chops topped with the mango salsa.

Prep Time: 15 minutes

Nutritional Value: Calories: 415, Fat: 20.2g, Saturated fat: 5.7g, Carbohydrates: 8.9g, Protein: 44.7g

15. Greek-Style Grilled Pork Kebabs
INGREDIENTS:
- - 2 tablespoons olive oil
- - 2 tablespoons freshly squeezed lemon juice
- - 2 cloves garlic, minced
- - 1 teaspoon dried oregano

- - 1 teaspoon ground cumin
- - 1 teaspoon smoked paprika
- - 1 pound pork tenderloin, cut into cubes
- - 1 red onion, cut into cubes
- - 1/2 teaspoon freshly ground black pepper
- - 1/2 teaspoon salt

Cooking Method:
1. In a small bowl, mix together the olive oil, lemon juice, garlic, oregano, cumin, and smoked paprika.
2. Place the pork cubes and red onion cubes in a shallow dish and pour the marinade over them.
3. Cover and refrigerate for at least 1 hour.
4. Preheat the grill or grill pan to medium-high heat.
5. Thread the pork and onion onto skewers and season with the black pepper and salt.

6. Grill the kebabs for 8 minutes, turning them occasionally, or until cooked through.
7. Serve hot.

Prep Time: 1 hour and 10 minutes
Nutritional Value: Calories: 260, Fat: 13.7g, Saturated fat: 3.2g, Carbohydrates: 4.4g, Protein: 29.4g

CHAPTER 6: STAPLES AND SWEETS RECIPES FOR BLOOD PRESSURE DOWN

1. Overnight Oats
INGREDIENTS:
- ½ cup of rolled oats
- ½ cup of almond milk
- ½ cup of plain Greek yogurt
- 1 teaspoon of honey
- 1 teaspoon of chia seeds
- ½ teaspoon of ground cinnamon
- Fresh fruit of choice

Cooking Method:
1. In a medium bowl, combine the rolled oats, almond milk, Greek yogurt, honey, chia seeds, and ground cinnamon.
2. Mix all the INGREDIENTS together until they are well combined.

3. Place the mixture in a jar or a container with a lid.
4. Place it in the refrigerator for at least 4 hours, or overnight.
5. Serve with fresh fruit of choice.

Prep Time: 10 minutes
Nutrition Value (per serving): Calories: 172, Fat: 4.7g, Carbohydrates: 25.5g, Protein: 7.7g

2. Baked Sweet Potato Fries
INGREDIENTS:
- 2 large sweet potatoes
- 2 tablespoons of olive oil
- 1 teaspoon of garlic powder
- 1 teaspoon of paprika
- ½ teaspoon of black pepper

Cooking Method:
1. Preheat the oven to 425 degrees F.

2. Peel the sweet potatoes and cut them into thin fry shapes.
3. Place the sweet potato fries onto a baking sheet.
4. Drizzle with the olive oil and sprinkle with the garlic powder, paprika, and black pepper.
5. Toss the fries until they are evenly coated.
6. Bake for 30 minutes, or until the fries are golden brown and crispy.

Prep Time: 20 minutes
Nutrition Value (per serving): Calories: 225, Fat: 10.4g, Carbohydrates: 30.4g, Protein: 2.4g

3. Pesto Salmon
INGREDIENTS:
- 2 salmon filets
- 2 tablespoons of pesto

- 2 tablespoons of olive oil
- 2 tablespoons of lemon juice
- 1 teaspoon of garlic powder
- 1 teaspoon of dried oregano

Cooking Method:
1. Preheat the oven to 375 degrees F.
2. Place the salmon filets onto a baking sheet.
3. In a small bowl, combine the pesto, olive oil, lemon juice, garlic powder, and dried oregano.
4. Spread the pesto mixture over the salmon filets.
5. Bake for 15-20 minutes, or until the salmon is cooked through.

Prep Time: 25 minutes
Nutrition Value (per serving): Calories: 279, Fat: 19.2g, Carbohydrates: 2.4g, Protein: 24.4g

4. Quinoa and Black Bean Salad

INGREDIENTS:

- 1 cup of cooked quinoa
- 1 can of black beans, drained and rinsed
- 1 red bell pepper, diced
- 1 cup of corn
- 2 green onions, diced
- ½ cup of cilantro, chopped
- 2 tablespoons of olive oil
- 2 tablespoons of freshly squeezed lime juice

Cooking Method:

1. In a large bowl, combine the cooked quinoa, black beans, red bell pepper, corn, green onions, and cilantro.
2. Drizzle with the olive oil and lime juice and mix until everything is well combined.
3. Serve chilled or at room temperature.

Prep Time: 15 minutes
Nutrition Value (per serving): Calories: 291, Fat: 8.3g, Carbohydrates: 45.3g, Protein: 10.3g

5. Roasted Vegetable Bowl

INGREDIENTS:

- 2 sweet potatoes, cut into cubes
- 2 zucchini, cut into cubes
- 1 red bell pepper, diced
- 1 onion, diced
- 2 tablespoons of olive oil
- 1 teaspoon of garlic powder
- 1 teaspoon of dried oregano
- ½ teaspoon of black pepper

Cooking Method:
1. Preheat the oven to 400 degrees F.
2. Place the sweet potato cubes, zucchini cubes, red bell pepper, and onion onto a baking sheet.

3. Drizzle with the olive oil and sprinkle with the garlic powder, oregano, and black pepper.
4. Toss the vegetables until they are evenly coated.
5. Bake for 25-30 minutes, or until the vegetables are tender and lightly browned.

Prep Time: 20 minutes
Nutrition Value (per serving): Calories: 343, Fat: 9.7g, Carbohydrates: 57.2g, Protein: 7.2g

6. Avocado Toast

INGREDIENTS:

- 2 slices of whole-grain bread
- 1 avocado, mashed
- 1 tablespoon of olive oil
- 1 teaspoon of freshly squeezed lemon juice

- 1 teaspoon of garlic powder
- 1 teaspoon of paprika
- Salt and pepper to taste

Cooking Method:
1. Toast the bread slices until golden brown.
2. In a small bowl, mash the avocado with a fork.
3. Mix in the olive oil, lemon juice, garlic powder, paprika, salt, and pepper.
4. Spread the mashed avocado mixture over the toasted bread slices.

Prep Time: 10 minutes
Nutrition Value (per serving): Calories: 153, Fat: 10.1g, Carbohydrates: 15.3g, Protein: 3.1g

7. Grilled Chicken Breast
INGREDIENTS:

- 2 chicken breasts
- 2 tablespoons of olive oil
- 1 teaspoon of garlic powder
- 1 teaspoon of paprika
- ½ teaspoon of black pepper

Cooking Method:
1. Preheat the grill to medium-high heat.
2. Rub the chicken breasts with the olive oil and sprinkle with the garlic powder, paprika, and black pepper.
3. Place the chicken breasts on the preheated grill.
4. Grill for 8-10 minutes, flipping halfway through, or until the chicken is cooked through.

Prep Time: 10 minutes
Nutrition Value (per serving): Calories: 227, Fat: 12.6g, Carbohydrates: 0.4g, Protein: 28.6g

8. Greek Yogurt Parfait

INGREDIENTS:

- ½ cup of plain Greek yogurt
- ¼ cup of granola
- 2 tablespoons of chopped walnuts
- 2 tablespoons of raisins
- 2 tablespoons of honey

Cooking Method:

1. In a small bowl, layer the Greek yogurt, granola, walnuts, and raisins.
2. Drizzle with the honey.
3. Serve chilled.

Prep Time: 5 minutes
Nutrition Value (per serving): Calories: 228, Fat: 8.1g, Carbohydrates: 31.6g, Protein: 7.1g

9. Lentil and Mushroom Stew

INGREDIENTS:

- 1 tablespoon of olive oil
- 1 onion, diced
- 2 cloves of garlic, minced
- 2 carrots, diced
- 2 celery stalks, diced
- 8 ounces of mushrooms, sliced
- 1 cup of green lentils, uncooked
- 4 cups of vegetable broth
- 1 teaspoon of dried thyme
- ½ teaspoon of black pepper

Cooking Method:

1. Heat the olive oil in a large pot over medium heat.
2. Add the onion, garlic, carrots, and celery and sauté for 5 minutes.
3. Add the mushrooms and continue to sauté for another 5 minutes.

4. Add the lentils, vegetable broth, thyme, and black pepper to the pot and bring it to a boil.

5. Reduce the heat and simmer for 25 minutes, or until the lentils are tender.

Prep Time: 25 minutes
Nutrition Value (per serving): Calories: 239, Fat: 5.3g, Carbohydrates: 36.3g, Protein: 12.2g

10. Grilled Fish Tacos

INGREDIENTS:

- 2 salmon filets
- 2 tablespoons of olive oil
- 2 teaspoons of garlic powder
- 2 teaspoons of paprika
- 1 teaspoon of dried oregano
- 6 small flour tortillas
- 1 cup of shredded cabbage
- ½ cup of diced tomatoes

- 2 limes, cut into wedges

Cooking Method:
1. Preheat the grill to medium-high heat.
2. Rub the salmon filets with the olive oil and sprinkle with the garlic powder, paprika, and oregano.
3. Place the salmon filets onto the preheated grill.
4. Grill for 8-10 minutes, flipping halfway through, or until the salmon is cooked through.
5. Slice the salmon into strips and assemble the tacos with the salmon, tortillas, cabbage, tomatoes, and limes.

Prep Time: 25 minutes
Nutrition Value (per serving): Calories: 324, Fat: 14.7g, Carbohydrates: 29.2g, Protein: 18.2g

11. Broccoli and Chickpea Curry

INGREDIENTS:

- 2 tablespoons olive oil
- 1 onion, finely chopped
- 4 garlic cloves, minced
- 1 teaspoon ground cumin
- 1 teaspoon ground coriander
- 1 teaspoon ground turmeric
- 1 teaspoon ground ginger
- 1/2 teaspoon chili powder
- 2 cups vegetable broth
- 1 can (14.5 ounces) diced tomatoes
- 2 cups cooked chickpeas
- 2 cups chopped broccoli florets
- 1/2 cup coconut milk
- Fresh cilantro leaves, for garnish

Cooking Method:

1. Heat the oil in a large skillet over medium heat. Add the onion and garlic and cook, stirring, until the onion is softened, about 5 minutes.

2. Add the cumin, coriander, turmeric, ginger, and chili powder and cook, stirring, for 1 minute.

3. Add the vegetable broth, tomatoes, chickpeas, and broccoli and bring to a simmer.

4. Reduce the heat to low and simmer, stirring occasionally, until the broccoli is tender, about 10 minutes.
5. Stir in the coconut milk and cook for a few minutes more.
6. Garnish with cilantro and serve.

Prep Time: 10 minutes
Cook Time: 20 minutes
Nutritional Value: Calories: 276, Total Fat: 11g, Saturated Fat: 3g, Cholesterol: 0mg, Sodium: 471mg, Total Carbohydrates: 33g, Dietary Fiber: 9g, Sugars: 8g, Protein: 11g

12. Veggie Burger

INGREDIENTS:

- 1/2 cup cooked brown rice
- 1/2 cup cooked quinoa
- 1/2 cup cooked black beans
- 1/2 cup grated zucchini
- 1/4 cup rolled oats
- 2 tablespoons chopped fresh parsley
- 1 tablespoon ground flaxseeds
- 1 teaspoon smoked paprika
- 1 teaspoon garlic powder
- 1/2 teaspoon ground cumin
- 2 tablespoons olive oil
- 4 whole wheat hamburger buns
- Lettuce, tomato, and onion, as desired

Cooking Method:

1. Preheat the oven to 375°F.

2. In a large bowl, combine the brown rice, quinoa, black beans, zucchini, oats, parsley, flaxseeds, paprika, garlic powder, and cumin. Mix well.

3. Form the mixture into 4 patties.

4. Heat the oil in a large oven-safe skillet over medium-high heat. Add the patties and cook for 4 minutes on each side, or until golden brown.

5. Transfer the skillet to the oven and bake for 15 minutes, or until cooked through.

6. Meanwhile, warm the buns in the oven.

7. Assemble the burgers on the buns with lettuce, tomato, and onion.

Prep Time: 10 minutes

Cook Time: 25 minutes
Nutritional Value: Calories: 364, Total
Fat: 9g, Saturated Fat: 1g, Cholesterol:
0mg, Sodium: 270mg, Total
Carbohydrates: 59g, Dietary Fiber: 10g,
Sugars: 5g, Protein: 11g

13. Zucchini Noodles

INGREDIENTS:

- 2 tablespoons olive oil
- 2 cloves garlic, minced
- 2 large zucchinis, spiralized
- 1/4 teaspoon red pepper flakes
- 2 tablespoons chopped fresh basil
- 2 tablespoons grated Parmesan cheese

Cooking Method:
1. Heat the oil in a large skillet over medium heat. Add the garlic and cook, stirring, until fragrant, about 30 seconds.

2. Add the zucchini noodles and red pepper flakes and cook, stirring, until the noodles are just tender, about 5 minutes.

3. Remove from the heat and stir in the basil and Parmesan.

Prep Time: 5 minutes
Cook Time: 10 minutes
Nutritional Value: Calories: 132, Total Fat: 10g, Saturated Fat: 2g, Cholesterol: 4mg, Sodium: 57mg, Total Carbohydrates: 8g, Dietary Fiber: 2g, Sugars: 5g, Protein: 4g

14. Kale Salad
INGREDIENTS:
- 1 bunch kale, chopped
- 2 tablespoons olive oil
- 1 tablespoon lemon juice

- 1/4 cup toasted walnuts
- 1/4 cup dried cranberries
- 1/4 cup crumbled feta cheese

Cooking Method:
1. In a large bowl, combine the kale, olive oil, and lemon juice and toss to coat.

2. Add the walnuts, cranberries, and feta cheese and toss to combine.

Prep Time: 10 minutes
Cook Time: 0 minutes
Nutritional Value: Calories: 191, Total Fat: 13g, Saturated Fat: 3g, Cholesterol: 10mg, Sodium: 163 mg, Total Carbohydrates: 15g, Dietary Fiber: 2g, Sugars: 7g, Protein: 6g

15. Lentil and Brown Rice Soup

INGREDIENTS:

- 2 tablespoons olive oil
- 1 onion, chopped
- 2 carrots, chopped
- 2 celery stalks, chopped
- 2 cloves garlic, minced
- 1 teaspoon dried thyme
- 1 teaspoon dried oregano
- 6 cups vegetable broth
- 1 cup dry lentils
- 1/2 cup dry brown rice
- 1 bay leaf
- 1/4 teaspoon black pepper

Cooking Method:

1. Heat the oil in a large pot over medium heat. Add the onion, carrots, celery, and garlic and cook, stirring, until the vegetables are softened, about 5 minutes.

2. Add the thyme and oregano and cook, stirring, for 1 minute.

3. Add the vegetable broth, lentils, rice, bay leaf, and black pepper and bring to a simmer.

4. Reduce the heat to low and simmer, stirring occasionally, until the lentils and rice are tender, about 45 minutes.

5. Remove the bay leaf before serving.

Prep Time: 10 minutes
Cook Time: 55 minutes
Nutritional Value: Calories: 305, Total Fat: 7g, Saturated Fat: 1g, Cholesterol: 0mg, Sodium: 562 mg, Total Carbohydrates: 45g, Dietary Fiber: 16g, Sugars: 7g, Protein: 16g

16. Greek Salad

INGREDIENTS:

- 2 cups chopped romaine lettuce
- 1/2 cup sliced cucumber
- 1/2 cup cherry tomatoes, halved
- 1/2 cup sliced red onion
- 1/4 cup Kalamata olives
- 1/4 cup crumbled feta cheese
- 2 tablespoons olive oil
- 1 tablespoon red wine vinegar
- 1 teaspoon dried oregano

Cooking Method:

1. In a large bowl, combine the lettuce, cucumber, tomatoes, red onion, and olives.

2. Add the feta cheese, olive oil, vinegar, and oregano and toss to combine.

Prep Time: 10 minutes
Cook Time: 0 minutes

Nutritional Value: Calories: 213, Total Fat: 17g, Saturated Fat: 3g, Cholesterol: 9mg, Sodium: 389 mg, Total Carbohydrates: 12g, Dietary Fiber: 3g, Sugars: 5g, Protein: 5g

17. Roasted Cauliflower
INGREDIENTS:
- 1 head cauliflower, cut into florets
- 2 tablespoons olive oil
- 1 teaspoon garlic powder
- 1 teaspoon smoked paprika
- 1/2 teaspoon ground cumin
- 1/4 teaspoon black pepper

Cooking Method:
1. Preheat the oven to 400°F.

2. In a large bowl, combine the cauliflower, olive oil, garlic powder,

paprika, cumin, and black pepper and toss to coat.

3. Spread the cauliflower on a rimmed baking sheet and bake for 20 minutes, or until golden brown.

Prep Time: 5 minutes
Cook Time: 20 minutes
Nutritional Value: Calories: 140, Total Fat: 10g, Saturated Fat: 1g, Cholesterol: 0mg, Sodium: 55mg, Total Carbohydrates: 11g, Dietary Fiber: 5g, Sugars: 4g, Protein: 4g

18. Fruit Smoothie
INGREDIENTS:
- 1 banana, sliced
- 1 cup frozen strawberries
- 1/2 cup plain Greek yogurt
- 1/2 cup unsweetened almond milk

- 1 tablespoon honey

Cooking Method:
1. In a blender, combine the banana, strawberries, yogurt, almond milk, and honey and blend until smooth.

Prep Time: 5 minutes
Cook Time: 0 minutes
Nutritional Value: Calories: 186, Total Fat: 2g, Saturated Fat: 0g, Cholesterol: 3mg, Sodium: 79 mg, Total Carbohydrates: 34g, Dietary Fiber: 4g, Sugars: 25g, Protein: 9g

19. Apple Cinnamon Oatmeal
INGREDIENTS:
- 1 cup rolled oats
- 2 cups unsweetened almond milk
- 1 apple, cored and diced
- 1 teaspoon ground cinnamon

- 2 tablespoons honey

Cooking Method:
1. In a medium saucepan, combine the oats, almond milk, apple, and cinnamon and bring to a simmer.

2. Reduce the heat to low and simmer, stirring occasionally, until the oats are tender and most of the liquid is absorbed, about 10 minutes.

3. Remove from the heat and stir in the honey.

Prep Time: 5 minutes
Cook Time: 10 minutes
Nutritional Value: Calories: 310, Total Fat: 5g, Saturated Fat: 0g, Cholesterol: 0mg, Sodium: 80mg, Total Carbohydrates: 58g, Dietary Fiber: 8g, Sugars: 29g, Protein: 8g

20. Greek Yogurt with Berries

INGREDIENTS:

- 2 cups Greek yogurt
- 1/2 cup fresh blueberries
- 1/2 cup fresh raspberries
- 2 tablespoons honey

Cooking Method:

1. In a medium bowl, combine the yogurt, blueberries, and raspberries.

2. Drizzle with the honey and mix to combine.

Prep Time: 5 minutes
Cook Time: 0 minutes
Nutritional Value: Calories: 214, Total Fat: 4g, Saturated Fat: 2g, Cholesterol: 11mg, Sodium: 75mg, Total Carbohydrates: 32g, Dietary Fiber: 4g, Sugars: 23g, Protein: 14g

HOMEMADE BREADS AND CAKES RECIPES

1. Banana Oat Cake with Coconut Topping

INGREDIENTS:

- - 2 large ripe bananas
- - 1 cup oats
- - 2 tablespoons coconut oil
- - 1/2 teaspoon baking powder
- - 2 tablespoons brown sugar
- - 1/2 cup desiccated coconut
- - 2 tablespoons honey
- - 1 teaspoon vanilla extract

Cooking method:

1. Preheat the oven to 350 F.
2. In a medium bowl, mash the bananas until smooth.
3. Add the oats, coconut oil, baking powder, brown sugar, and desiccated coconut.

4. Mix together until fully combined.

5. Grease a 9-inch baking dish and spread the mixture evenly into the dish.

6. Bake for 20-25 minutes until golden brown.

7. Meanwhile, in a small bowl, mix together the honey, vanilla extract and desiccated coconut.

8. When the cake is done baking, spread the coconut mixture over the top.

9. Serve warm or at room temperature.

Prep Time: 15 minutes
Cook Time: 25 minutes
Nutritional Value: calories- 188, fat- 8.6g, carbohydrates- 27.2g, protein- 3.2g

2. Chocolate Avocado Cake

INGREDIENTS:
- - 2 ripe avocados
- - 2 cups almond flour

- - 1/4 cup cocoa powder
- - 2 teaspoons baking powder
- - 1/4 cup maple syrup
- - 2 tablespoons coconut oil
- - 1 teaspoon vanilla extract
- - 2 tablespoons dark chocolate chips

Cooking method:
1. Preheat the oven to 350 F.
2. Grease a 9-inch baking dish.
3. In a medium bowl, mash the avocados until smooth.
4. Add the almond flour, cocoa powder, baking powder, maple syrup, coconut oil, and vanilla extract.
5. Mix together until fully combined.
6. Spread the mixture evenly into the baking dish.
7. Sprinkle the chocolate chips over the top.
8. Bake for 25-30 minutes until golden brown.

Prep Time: 10 minutes
Cook Time: 30 minutes
Nutritional Value: calories- 293, fat- 19.7g, carbohydrates- 22.8g, protein- 8.9g

3. Apple Cinnamon Cake with Yogurt Frosting

INGREDIENTS:

- - 2 cups almond flour
- - 1 teaspoon baking powder
- - 2 teaspoons ground cinnamon
- - 2 tablespoons coconut oil
- - 1/4 cup applesauce
- - 1/4 cup maple syrup
- - 1 teaspoon vanilla extract
- - 2 apples, cored and diced
- - For the frosting:
- - 1/2 cup Greek yogurt
- - 2 tablespoons honey

Cooking method:
1. Preheat the oven to 350 F.
2. Grease a 9-inch baking dish.
3. In a medium bowl, mix together the almond flour, baking powder and ground cinnamon.
4. Add the coconut oil, applesauce, maple syrup and vanilla extract.
5. Mix until fully combined.
6. Fold in the apples.
7. Spread the mixture evenly into the baking dish.
8. Bake for 25-30 minutes until golden brown.
9. Meanwhile, in a small bowl, mix together the yogurt and honey.
10. Spread the yogurt frosting over the top of the cake.
11. Serve warm or at room temperature.

Prep Time: 10 minutes
Cook Time: 30 minutes

Nutritional Value: calories- 255, fat-13.3g, carbohydrates- 26.2g, protein-8.3g

4. Zucchini Carrot Cake
INGREDIENTS:
- - 2 cups almond flour
- - 1 teaspoon baking powder
- - 1/4 teaspoon ground cinnamon
- - 2 tablespoons coconut oil
- - 1/4 cup maple syrup
- - 1 teaspoon vanilla extract
- - 1 cup grated zucchini
- - 1 cup grated carrot

Cooking method:
1. Preheat the oven to 350 F.
2. Grease a 9-inch baking dish.
3. In a medium bowl, mix together the almond flour, baking powder and ground cinnamon.

4. Add the coconut oil, maple syrup and vanilla extract.

5. Mix until fully combined.

6. Fold in the zucchini and carrots.

7. Spread the mixture evenly into the baking dish.

8. Bake for 25-30 minutes until golden brown.

Prep Time: 10 minutes
Cook Time: 30 minutes
Nutritional Value: calories- 227, fat- 12.3g, carbohydrates- 22.5g, protein- 7.1g

5. Hummingbird Cake
INGREDIENTS:
- - 2 cups almond flour
- - 1 teaspoon baking powder
- - 1/4 teaspoon ground cinnamon
- - 2 tablespoons coconut oil
- - 1/4 cup maple syrup

- - 1 teaspoon vanilla extract
- - 1 cup mashed banana
- - 1/2 cup crushed pineapple
- - 2 tablespoons chopped walnuts

Cooking method:
1. Preheat the oven to 350 F.
2. Grease a 9-inch baking dish.
3. In a medium bowl, mix together the almond flour, baking powder and ground cinnamon.
4. Add the coconut oil, maple syrup and vanilla extract.
5. Mix until fully combined.
6. Fold in the mashed banana, crushed pineapple and walnuts.
7. Spread the mixture evenly into the baking dish.
8. Bake for 25-30 minutes until golden brown.

Prep Time: 10 minutes
Cook Time: 30 minutes

Nutritional Value: calories- 235, fat-
11.6g, carbohydrates- 28.3g, protein- 7.1g

6. Date and Almond Cake

INGREDIENTS:

- - 2 cups almond flour
- - 1 teaspoon baking powder
- - 2 tablespoons coconut oil
- - 1/4 cup maple syrup
- - 1 teaspoon vanilla extract
- - 1 cup chopped dates
- - 1/2 cup chopped almonds

Cooking method:

1. Preheat the oven to 350 F.
2. Grease a 9-inch baking dish.
3. In a medium bowl, mix together the almond flour, baking powder and ground cinnamon.
4. Add the coconut oil, maple syrup and vanilla extract.

5. Mix until fully combined.
6. Fold in the chopped dates and almonds.
7. Spread the mixture evenly into the baking dish.
8. Bake for 25-30 minutes until golden brown.

Prep Time: 10 minutes
Cook Time: 30 minutes
Nutritional Value: calories- 271, fat- 15.2g, carbohydrates- 27.8g, protein- 8.0g

7. Blueberry Almond Cake
INGREDIENTS:
- - 2 cups almond flour
- - 1 teaspoon baking powder
- - 2 tablespoons coconut oil
- - 1/4 cup maple syrup
- - 1 teaspoon vanilla extract

- - 1/2 cup blueberries
- - 1/2 cup chopped almonds

Cooking method:
1. Preheat the oven to 350 F.
2. Grease a 9-inch baking dish.
3. In a medium bowl, mix together the almond flour, baking powder and ground cinnamon.
4. Add the coconut oil, maple syrup and vanilla extract.
5. Mix until fully combined.
6. Fold in the blueberries and almonds.
7. Spread the mixture evenly into the baking dish.
8. Bake for 25-30 minutes until golden brown.

Prep Time: 10 minutes
Cook Time: 30 minutes
Nutritional Value: calories- 287, fat- 16.4g, carbohydrates- 25.7g, protein- 8.3g

8. Orange and Almond Flour Cake
INGREDIENTS:
- - 2 cups almond flour
- - 1 teaspoon baking powder
- - 2 tablespoons coconut oil
- - 1/4 cup maple syrup
- - 1 teaspoon vanilla extract
- - 1/2 cup freshly squeezed orange juice
- - 2 tablespoons chopped almonds

Cooking method:
1. Preheat the oven to 350 F.
2. Grease a 9-inch baking dish.
3. In a medium bowl, mix together the almond flour, baking powder and ground cinnamon.
4. Add the coconut oil, maple syrup, vanilla extract and orange juice.
5. Mix until fully combined.

6. Fold in the almonds.

7. Spread the mixture evenly into the baking dish.

8. Bake for 25-30 minutes until golden brown.

Prep Time: 10 minutes

Cook Time: 30 minutes

Nutritional Value: calories- 207, fat- 11.6g, carbohydrates- 19.4g, protein- 7.4g

9. Quinoa Chocolate Cake

INGREDIENTS:

- - 1 cup cooked quinoa
- - 1/2 cup almond flour
- - 1/4 cup cocoa powder
- - 2 teaspoons baking powder
- - 2 tablespoons coconut oil
- - 1/4 cup maple syrup
- - 1 teaspoon vanilla extract
- - 2 tablespoons dark chocolate chips

Cooking method:
1. Preheat the oven to 350 F.
2. Grease a 9-inch baking dish.
3. In a medium bowl, mash the cooked quinoa until smooth.
4. Add the almond flour, cocoa powder, baking powder, coconut oil, maple syrup and vanilla extract.
5. Mix together until fully combined.
6. Spread the mixture evenly into the baking dish.
7. Sprinkle the chocolate chips over the top.
8. Bake for 25-30 minutes until golden brown.

Prep Time: 10 minutes
Cook Time: 30 minutes
Nutritional Value: calories- 290, fat- 13.8g, carbohydrates- 35.2g, protein- 7.8g

CHAPTER 7: HEALTHY COOKING TECHNIQUES FOR HIGH BLOOD PRESSURE

1. Use Healthy Fats: Use healthy fats such as olive oil, canola oil and other unsaturated fats in place of saturated fats such as butter and lard.

2. Grill, Bake, Broil, or Stir-Fry: When cooking, choose methods that use little or no added fat such as grilling, baking, broiling, or stir-frying.

3. Cut Back on Salt: When cooking and eating, reduce the amount of salt used. Instead, use herbs and spices to add flavor to your food.

4. Eat More Fiber: Add more fiber to your diet by eating more fruits, vegetables, and whole grains.

5. Choose Lean Meats: Choose lean meats such as chicken, fish, and turkey. Trim away visible fat before cooking.

6. Use Low-Fat Dairy Products: Choose low-fat or non-fat dairy products such as milk, yogurt, and cheese.

7. Limit Alcohol: Limit your alcohol intake to no more than one or two drinks per day.

BLOOD PRESSURE FLAVOR-ENHANCING STRATEGIES WITHOUT ADDED SODIUM

1. Spice It Up: Use herbs and spices such as garlic, cumin, paprika, oregano, and cinnamon to add flavor to food.

2. Add Acidity: Try adding citrus juices like lemon, lime, or orange to dishes. Vinegars like balsamic, red wine, and apple cider also add a tart flavor.

3. Experiment with Herbs: Fresh herbs like basil, rosemary, thyme, and parsley can be used to liven up dishes.

4. Incorporate Fruits: Fruits like apples, oranges, and cranberries can add sweetness and flavor to dishes.

5. Try Fats: Adding healthy fats like olive oil, avocado, or nuts can help round out flavors.

6. Get Saucy: Use low-sodium sauces like salsa or pesto to add flavor to dishes.

7. Get Creative: Try adding interesting ingredients like capers, olives, or mushrooms to dishes.

BLOOD PRESSURE AND OTHER HEALTH CONDITIONS

How is Blood Pressure linked to the below Health Conditions Health Conditions?.
   1. DIABETES
   2. KIDNEY DISEASE

3. HEART DISEASE
4. OBESITY

Blood pressure is an important indicator of overall health and is a key risk factor for several serious health conditions. High blood pressure, also known as hypertension, is particularly dangerous because it can cause a variety of problems throughout the body. It is linked to a number of conditions including diabetes, kidney disease, heart disease, and obesity.

Diabetes is a condition in which the body does not properly regulate blood sugar levels. When blood sugar levels are too high, the body's cells become resistant to insulin, a hormone produced by the pancreas that helps regulate blood sugar levels. This resistance can cause high blood pressure, as the body is unable to properly process glucose, resulting in higher levels of glucose and other substances that increase blood pressure. Additionally, people with diabetes are more likely to be obese and have other conditions, such as high cholesterol, that can also contribute to high blood pressure.

Kidney disease is a condition in which the kidneys are unable to filter waste and excess fluids from the body. As a result, the body retains more fluid, resulting in an increase in blood volume and pressure. People with kidney disease are also more likely to have high cholesterol, which can further contribute to high blood pressure.

Heart disease is a condition in which the heart is unable to pump blood efficiently. This can lead to an increase in blood pressure as the heart must work harder to pump blood throughout the body. In addition, people with heart disease may also have high cholesterol, which can contribute to high blood pressure.

Obesity is a condition in which a person has an excessive amount of body fat. This can lead to high blood pressure due to increased levels of fat and cholesterol in the bloodstream. Additionally, obesity can lead to an increase in insulin resistance, which can further contribute to high blood pressure.

BLOOD PRESSURE DIET ON A BUDGET

MEAL PLANNING TIPS

1. Increase your intake of fruits and vegetables. Fruits and vegetables are high

in vitamins, minerals, and fiber, and are generally low in calories and fat. Eating a variety of fruits and vegetables can help to reduce blood pressure.

2. Eat foods rich in potassium. Foods such as bananas, spinach, potatoes, and sweet potatoes are high in potassium, which can help to reduce high blood pressure.

3. Choose lean proteins. Lean proteins such as fish, chicken, or turkey can help to reduce high blood pressure.

4. Limit sodium intake. Sodium can cause your body to retain fluid, which can increase your blood pressure. Try to limit your sodium intake to 2,300 milligrams per day.

5. Choose whole grain foods. Whole grain foods are high in fiber, which can help reduce high blood pressure.

6. Avoid processed foods. Processed foods are often high in sodium and low in nutrients, which can contribute to high blood pressure.

7. Avoid added sugars. Added sugars can cause your body to retain fluid and can contribute to high blood pressure.

8. Drink alcohol in moderation. Drinking too much alcohol can cause your blood pressure to increase. Limit your alcohol intake to normal.

STRESS MANAGEMENT FOR LOWERING BLOOD PRESSURE

Stress management is an important tool for reducing high blood pressure. Stress can cause your body to produce hormones that constrict your blood vessels, raising your blood pressure. To help reduce your stress and lower your blood pressure, here are some tips:

1. Exercise: Regular physical activity can help reduce stress and lower your blood pressure. Exercise can also help you manage your weight and maintain healthy cholesterol levels.

2. Relaxation techniques: Deep breathing, meditation, and yoga are all effective ways to reduce stress and lower your blood pressure.

3. Healthy lifestyle: Eating a healthy diet, getting enough sleep, and limiting alcohol and caffeine consumption can all help reduce stress and lower your blood pressure.

4. Reduce stressors: Identifying and addressing the sources of your stress can help reduce your overall stress levels and lower your blood pressure.

5. Talk to someone: Talking with a trusted friend, family member, or mental health professional can help you find ways to manage your stress and lower your blood pressure.

EXERCISE FOR LOWERING BLOOD PRESSURE

1. Aerobic Exercise: Aerobic exercise, such as walking, biking, running, swimming, or dancing, increases heart rate and breathing. This helps to lower blood pressure by improving circulation and strengthening the heart.

2. Resistance Exercise: Resistance exercises, such as weight lifting, push ups, or squats, increase muscle strength and can help reduce blood pressure. This is because stronger muscles can help the heart work more efficiently.

3. Yoga and Stretching: Yoga and stretching exercises help relax the body

and reduce tension, which can help lower blood pressure.

4. Deep Breathing Exercises: Deep breathing exercises help relax the body and reduce stress, which can help to lower blood pressure.

5. Tai Chi: Tai chi is a form of meditation that combines movement and breathing. This exercise can help reduce stress and improve relaxation, which can help to lower blood pressure.

6. Meditation: Meditation can help to reduce stress, which can help to lower blood pressure.

7. Walking: Walking is a low-impact exercise that can help to improve circulation and reduce stress, which can help to lower blood pressure.

8. Cycling: Cycling is a low-impact exercise that can help to improve circulation and reduce stress, which can help to lower blood pressure.

SUPPLEMENTS FOR LOWERING BLOOD PRESSURE

There are several supplements that have been shown to potentially lower blood pressure, but it's important to note that these supplements should not be used as a substitute for medical treatment prescribed by a doctor.

Here are a few supplements that may help lower blood pressure:

Fish Oil: Fish oil can help reduce blood pressure by increasing the amount of omega-3 fatty acids in your diet, which can help reduce inflammation and lower triglyceride levels.

Omega-3 fatty acids: Found in fish oil supplements, these fatty acids have been shown to have a modest effect on reducing blood pressure.

Coenzyme Q10 (CoQ10): This antioxidant is found in every cell of the body and is involved in energy production. Some studies suggest that taking CoQ10 supplements may help lower blood pressure.

Garlic: Garlic supplements have been found to have a modest effect on reducing blood pressure in people with hypertension.

Magnesium: Magnesium supplements have been shown to have a small but significant effect on reducing blood pressure.

Potassium: Potassium supplements have been found to help lower blood pressure, especially in people with high salt intake.

Hibiscus: Some studies suggest that drinking hibiscus tea or taking hibiscus supplements may help lower blood pressure.

Hawthorn: Hawthorn is an herb that may improve blood vessel function and reduce blood pressure.

Vitamin C: Vitamin C can help reduce oxidative stress and lower blood pressure.

Danshen: Danshen is an herb that can help relax your blood vessels and lower blood pressure.

CONCLUSION

Frequently Asked Questions And Answers About Blood Pressure

QUESTION: What is the normal blood pressure (BP) range?

ANSWER:
Your blood pressure can change every minute. It can go up or down depending on your body position, breathing rhythm, stress level, activity level, and even the time of day. A normal blood pressure level is less than 120/80 mmHg (less than 120 systolic AND less than 80 diastolic). This can vary slightly depending on your age.

QUESTION: What is hypotension?

ANSWER:
Hypotension is a condition where the blood pressure is lower than normal, in this case; less than 90/60 mm Hg.

QUESTION: What are high and low blood pressure symptoms?

ANSWER:
A few symptoms of high blood pressure:

Dizziness
Shortness of breath
Headaches
Blurred vision
Nosebleeds(epistaxis)
Rapid or irregular heartbeat
(palpitations)
Nausea

Vomiting

A few symptoms of low blood pressure:

Light-headedness

Dizziness

Fainting (syncope)

Confusion

Blurring of vision

Nausea

Fatigue

QUESTION: What is considered high blood pressure?

ANSWER:
High blood pressure is defined as a blood pressure reading that is greater than 140/90 mmHg. A blood pressure reading of 130/80 mmHg is considered high, while a reading of 120/70 mmHg is considered moderate. Elevated blood

pressure can lead to heart disease, stroke, and other serious health problems.

QUESTION: What are the risks of having high blood pressure?

ANSWER:
There are many risks associated with high blood pressure, including heart disease, stroke, and kidney disease.

High blood pressure can also lead to vision problems, hearing loss, and difficulty breathing. If left untreated, high blood pressure can also lead to a heart attack or stroke.

There are many risks associated with high blood pressure, including heart disease, stroke, and kidney failure. If left untreated, high blood pressure can lead to a heart attack or stroke.

High blood pressure is a major risk factor for heart disease, stroke, and other serious health problems. It can also lead to kidney failure, blindness, and other serious complications. If you have high blood pressure, you should see your doctor as soon as possible to get it under control. There are many ways to lower your blood pressure, including medication, diet, and exercise.

QUESTION: What can I do to lower my blood pressure?

ANSWER:
There are many things you can do to lower your blood pressure. Some of the most common include eating a healthy

diet, getting regular exercise, and avoiding smoking. You can also take medications to lower your blood pressure.

QUESTION: Which arm is used to take blood pressure readings?

ANSWER:
Most people take blood pressure readings with their left arm. However, people with certain medical conditions or who have had a stroke may need to take blood pressure readings with the right arm.

QUESTION: When is the best time to take my blood pressure medication?

ANSWER:

There is no definitive answer to this question. Some people prefer to take their blood pressure medication Drugs for High Blood Pressure at bedtime, while others feel that it is more effective to take the medication in the morning. Ultimately, it is up to the individual to decide when they feel the best taking their blood pressure medication.

QUESTION: How do I take my blood pressure?

ANSWER:
There are a few ways to lower your blood pressure. One way is to use a sphygmomanometer, which is a simple, inexpensive device that you can buy at most pharmacies. You can also use an automated blood pressure monitor, which is a more accurate way to measure

your blood pressure, but it is more expensive. You can also ask your doctor to measure your blood pressure.

QUESTION:
Can alcohol increase blood pressure?

ANSWER:
Yes, alcohol can increase blood pressure. Drinking alcohol can increase your heart rate and cause your blood pressure to rise. Alcohol can also cause your blood vessels to constrict, which can lead to high blood pressure.

QUESTION: What is the best exercise to lower blood pressure?

ANSWER:

There is no one-size-fits-all answer to this question, as the best exercise to lower blood pressure will vary depending on your individual health and fitness level. However, some general recommendations for reducing blood pressure include:

Walking or jogging: These activities are relatively low-impact and can help to improve your overall fitness level.

Strength training: It can help to improve your overall strength and cardiovascular health, which can in turn help to lower your blood pressure,
And more...

QUESTION: When is high blood pressure an emergency?

ANSWER:

High blood pressure is a serious medical condition that can lead to heart disease, stroke, and even death. If you experience any of the following signs and symptoms, it is important to see a doctor: chest pain, shortness of breath, rapid heartbeat, sweating, nausea, or vomiting.

If high blood pressure is not treated, it can lead to heart attack, stroke, and even death. High blood pressure is considered an emergency if it causes any of the following: chest pain that does not go away, difficulty breathing, fainting, or blacking out.

QUESTION: Does high blood pressure cause headaches?

ANSWER:

There is some evidence that high blood pressure may cause headaches. Some people with high blood pressure may experience more frequent and severe headaches than people with lower blood pressure. High blood pressure may also increase the risk of other conditions that can cause headaches, such as stroke, heart disease, and dementia.

QUESTION: Is High Blood Pressure Curable?

ANSWER:

There is currently no cure for high blood pressure, but there are many ways to lower it. Treatment usually includes lifestyle changes (like losing weight), medication (like angiotensin-converting enzyme inhibitors or angiotensin receptor blockers), and surgery (like a heart valve replacement).

Some people can lower their blood pressure with diet and exercise alone. If you have high blood pressure, your doctor will want to do a blood test to see if you have the condition and if you need treatment.

QUESTION: Which blood pressure number is more important?

ANSWER:
The most important blood pressure number is systolic pressure, which is the top number in a blood pressure reading. The reason for this is that a higher systolic pressure indicates greater heart muscle activity and indicates a greater risk for heart problems.

QUESTION: Does smoking cause high blood pressure?

ANSWER:
Smoking has been linked with an increased risk of high blood pressure. Smoking is one of the most significant risk factors for developing high blood pressure. Smoking causes the body to produce more inflammation, which can lead to an increase in blood pressure.

Additionally, smoking can increase the risk of heart disease, stroke, and other cardiovascular problems. If you are concerned about your blood pressure, it is important to quit smoking and to make lifestyle changes that may help to lower your blood pressure.

QUESTION:
How long does it take blood pressure medicine to work?

ANSWER:
Blood pressure medicine works in two ways: by reducing the amount of blood that flows through your veins and by reducing the amount of blood that your heart has to pump. It can take up to several weeks for blood pressure medicine to work to its full effect.

QUESTION:
How does high blood pressure make you feel?

ANSWER:
High blood pressure can make you feel like you're having a heart attack, and it can also lead to other health problems. High blood pressure can cause you to

have a harder time breathing, and it can also lead to stroke, heart failure, and kidney failure. If you have high blood pressure, you should see a doctor as soon as possible to get it under control.

QUESTION: Can anxiety cause high blood pressure?

ANSWER:
There is some evidence that anxiety may be a contributing factor to high blood pressure, as anxiety can increase heart rate and cortisol levels, both of which can increase blood pressure. Additionally, people with high blood pressure are more likely to have anxiety disorders.

QUESTION: Does marijuana lower blood pressure?

ANSWER:
There is limited research on the effects of
marijuana on blood pressure. Some
studies have found that people who use
marijuana have a lower blood pressure
than people who do not use marijuana.
However, other studies have not found a
link between marijuana use and lower
blood pressure. More research is needed
to determine the effects of marijuana on
blood pressure.

RECAP OF KEY POINTS

If you're really looking for a way to naturally reduce your blood pressure, then THE AMERICAN HEART ASSOCIATION BLOOD PRESSURE LOWERING DIET COOKBOOK will be the perfect solution. With the help of a diet rich in nutritious foods, you can decrease your risk of hypertension and improve your overall health. Here are some key points to keep in mind when following going on this healing journey:

• Eat a balanced diet: Eating a balanced diet that is low in salt and saturated fat, and high in fiber, fruits, vegetables, and whole grains can help to lower your blood pressure. Make sure to include plenty of fresh fruits and vegetables in your meals, as well as lean proteins, healthy fats, and whole grains.

• Reduce sodium: Sodium is a key factor in high blood pressure, and reducing your intake of processed and restaurant foods can help to lower it. Choose foods with little to no added salt, and look for reduced-sodium options when purchasing packaged foods.

• Increase potassium: Potassium is one of the most important minerals for keeping blood pressure in check. Try to include more potassium-rich foods in your meals, such as bananas, potatoes, tomatoes, and spinach.

• Exercise regularly: Exercise can help to lower your blood pressure, so make sure to get 30 minutes of moderate physical activity every day.

• Manage stress: Stress can raise your blood pressure, so it's important to find ways to manage it. Try yoga, meditation, and deep breathing exercises to help you relax.

• Monitor Your Blood Pressure: Regularly monitoring your blood pressure at home can help you identify any sudden changes that may need medical attention, check your blood pressure regularly at least once in 2 days.

Following the THE AMERICAN HEART ASSOCIATION BLOOD PRESSURE LOWERING DIET COOKBOOK will help you to lower your blood pressure naturally and improve your overall health.

Eating a balanced diet that is low in salt and saturated fat, and high in fiber, fruits, vegetables, and whole grains, reducing your sodium intake, increasing your potassium intake, exercising regularly, and managing stress can all help to keep your blood pressure in check. Take advantage of the recipes and tips in the THe American Heart Association Blood Pressure Lowering Diet Cookbook to help you get started on a healthier lifestyle.

FINAL THOUGHTS AND ENCOURAGEMENT

The American Heart Association Blood Pressure Lowering Diet Cookbook has provided a wealth of recipes and tips to help you lower your blood pressure.

By incorporating the information in this cookbook, you will definitely achieve a healthier lifestyle and enjoy the delicious, nutritious recipes. With a little effort and dedication, you can be able to live a healthier, happier you.

Thank you for reading and good luck on your journey to healthier blood pressure levels!

DON'T FORGET TO LEAVE A POSITIVE AND A FRIENDLY REVIEW

Made in the USA
Columbia, SC
28 June 2023

19626501R00230